Table of Contents

12

The Global Impact of Diabetes

Diabetes is one of the most prevalent and complex chronic diseases affecting millions of people worldwide. It has become a global health crisis, touching nearly every corner of the world, regardless of nationality, socioeconomic status, or age. The World Health Organization (WHO) estimates that over 460 million people worldwide are currently living with diabetes, and that number continues to rise at an alarming rate. With the growing prevalence of obesity, sedentary lifestyles, and aging populations, diabetes is no longer a condition that is confined to a specific demographic—every society must grapple with its social, economic, and healthcare implications.

In addition to its impact on individuals and families, diabetes places a significant strain on healthcare systems globally. The costs of diabetes treatment and management—ranging from medications and insulin therapies to hospital admissions and long-term care—are staggering. According to the International Diabetes Federation (IDF), the global cost of diabetes has reached over $850 billion annually, and this figure is expected to grow substantially as the number of diabetes diagnoses continues to climb.

The consequences of diabetes are not limited to the economic impact; the human toll is profound. The disease is a leading cause of disability and death worldwide, contributing to complications such as cardiovascular disease, kidney failure, vision loss, and nerve damage. For many, managing diabetes is a daily challenge, requiring constant vigilance, lifestyle adjustments, and often, a sense of emotional and mental resilience.

A Brief History of Diabetes

The story of diabetes is a long and fascinating one, stretching back thousands of years. The term "diabetes" was first coined in ancient Greece by the physician Aretaeus of Cappadocia around 150 CE, deriving from the Greek word siphon due to the frequent urination characteristic of the condition. The full name, Diabetes Mellitus, was later introduced in the early 19th century, with mellitus meaning "honey-sweet" in Latin, referencing the sweet taste of the urine due to the presence of excess glucose.

However, it wasn't until the early 20th century that diabetes began to be understood as a disease of insulin deficiency, thanks to the groundbreaking discovery of insulin in 1921 by Canadian researchers Frederick Banting and Charles Best. The discovery of insulin revolutionized the treatment of Type 1 diabetes, transforming it from a fatal disease into a manageable condition. Prior to this, individuals with Type 1 diabetes often died within months of diagnosis due to severe complications from uncontrolled blood sugar.

The discovery of insulin also paved the way for the development of more sophisticated management techniques, such as blood glucose monitoring and advanced medication. In recent decades, progress in diabetes care has been further propelled by the advent of technologies like continuous glucose monitors (CGMs), insulin pumps, and the use of digital tools to track blood sugar levels, diet, and physical activity.

Despite these advancements, however, the global prevalence of diabetes continues to rise. Type 2 diabetes, once thought to be a condition mainly affecting older adults, is now being diagnosed in younger populations, with increasing rates in children and adolescents due to the rise in obesity and sedentary lifestyles.

The Scope and Objectives of This Book

Diabetes Unlocked aims to provide a comprehensive, yet accessible, resource for anyone affected by diabetes—whether directly or indirectly. This book delves deeply into the science behind the disease, the different types of diabetes, and the practical steps individuals can take to manage and thrive with the condition. The goal is to shed light on the complexities of diabetes, offering a holistic view that integrates medical knowledge, lifestyle strategies, and emotional support.

This book is divided into several parts to guide readers through the various facets of diabetes:

1. **The Basics of Diabetes:** This section covers the fundamental science behind diabetes, including how the body processes sugar, the role of insulin, and the physiological differences between the various types of diabetes.

2. **Types of Diabetes:** A detailed exploration of the most common types of diabetes—Type 1, Type 2, and gestational diabetes—along with less common forms like LADA (Latent Autoimmune Diabetes in Adults) and MODY (Maturity-Onset Diabetes of the Young). Each chapter will examine how these conditions develop, their risk factors, and their unique treatment approaches.

3. **Diagnosis and Early Intervention:** Here, we will focus on how diabetes is diagnosed, the role of early detection, and how timely intervention can

make a world of difference in terms of managing the condition and preventing complications.

4. **Management Strategies:** This section provides practical, actionable advice for managing diabetes on a day-to-day basis. Topics such as medication, insulin therapy, exercise, nutrition, and stress management will be explored in-depth.

5. **Living with Diabetes:** It's one thing to manage the disease medically, but it's another to live a fulfilling life while doing so. This part of the book offers insights into maintaining mental and emotional well-being, finding support, and building a balanced lifestyle.

6. **The Future of Diabetes Care:** The final chapters look forward to the exciting innovations in diabetes research and treatment, including the role of technology, stem cell therapy, and even the potential for a cure. The future of diabetes care is bright, and we will explore the possibilities that lie ahead.

By offering a thorough and multidimensional approach, Diabetes Unlocked seeks to empower readers with the knowledge and tools they need to not only survive diabetes but to thrive with it. Whether you are newly diagnosed or have been living with diabetes for years, this book will provide valuable insights and practical tips for taking control of your health.

Who Should Read This Book?

This book is designed for anyone who has a stake in the understanding and management of diabetes. It is written with a broad audience in mind, from those who have been diagnosed with the condition to their families, caregivers, healthcare professionals, and even those who are simply looking to expand their understanding of this widespread disease.

- **Individuals Diagnosed with Diabetes:** If you have been diagnosed with Type 1, Type 2, or any other form of diabetes, this book is here to provide clarity and guide you through the complexities of managing the condition. It offers practical advice on how to live a full, healthy life, despite the challenges of diabetes.

- **Caregivers and Family Members:** Diabetes is not just an individual condition; it affects families as well. If you are caring for a loved one with diabetes, this book will help you better understand the disease, offer guidance on how to provide support, and ensure that the person you care for receives the best possible care.

- **Healthcare Professionals:** Whether you are a doctor, nurse, dietitian, or other healthcare provider, Diabetes Unlocked can serve as a comprehensive reference to enhance your understanding of the disease and provide you with additional tools for supporting patients in their journey with diabetes.

- **Anyone Interested in Understanding Diabetes:** If you're simply looking to gain a deeper understanding of diabetes, this book offers the most up-to-date information on the disease, including emerging treatments, cutting-edge research, and the latest in diabetes technology. Diabetes can be overwhelming and confusing, but it doesn't have to be a barrier to living a full and vibrant life. With the right knowledge and support, people with diabetes can lead healthy, active, and meaningful lives. Diabetes Unlocked is not just about managing a disease; it's about unlocking the potential for a better future, a future where people with diabetes are equipped to not only survive, but to thrive.

Welcome to Diabetes Unlocked. We hope this book becomes a trusted guide on your journey toward understanding, managing, and ultimately mastering diabetes in all its forms.

Chapter 1: What is Diabetes?

Diabetes is a chronic medical condition that occurs when the body is unable to effectively regulate blood sugar (glucose) levels. Glucose is the primary source of energy for the body's cells, and it is derived from the foods we eat, especially carbohydrates. The body relies on insulin, a hormone produced by the pancreas, to help cells absorb glucose from the bloodstream and use it for energy. In diabetes, this process is disrupted, leading to abnormally high levels of glucose in the blood, known as hyperglycemia.

While the underlying causes of diabetes can vary, the consequences are often similar: over time, uncontrolled high blood sugar can damage organs, tissues, and cells throughout the body, leading to a wide range of complications. Fortunately, with proper diagnosis, management, and lifestyle changes, individuals with diabetes can lead healthy and fulfilling lives. Understanding the basics of diabetes—its types, causes, and effects—lays the foundation for effective management and treatment.

What Happens in the Body During Diabetes?

To understand diabetes, it's important to first grasp the role of glucose and insulin in the body. When we eat, food is broken down into its basic components—carbohydrates, proteins, and fats. The carbohydrates in our food are converted into glucose, which then enters the bloodstream. In response, the pancreas releases insulin, a hormone that acts like a key, allowing glucose to enter the body's cells to be used as energy. Without insulin, glucose cannot effectively enter cells, causing it to build up in the bloodstream.

In a healthy individual, insulin helps maintain blood glucose levels within a normal range. When the system is functioning correctly, glucose levels rise after eating and then gradually decrease as insulin facilitates the absorption of glucose by cells. However, in diabetes, the process of insulin regulation is disrupted, resulting in either insufficient insulin production or an inability of the body to respond to insulin effectively.

The Different Types of Diabetes

There are several types of diabetes, each with its own causes, risk factors, and treatment approaches. The two most common types are Type 1 diabetes and Type 2 diabetes, but there are also less common forms, such as gestational diabetes, Latent Autoimmune Diabetes in Adults (LADA), and Maturity-Onset Diabetes of the Young (MODY). Understanding these types helps clarify how diabetes can manifest differently in individuals.

Type 1 Diabetes (T1D)

Type 1 diabetes is an autoimmune condition in which the body's immune system mistakenly attacks and destroys the insulin-producing beta cells in the pancreas. This leaves individuals with Type 1 diabetes with little to no ability to produce insulin. Type 1 diabetes is typically diagnosed in childhood or adolescence, although it can occur at any age. The exact cause of this autoimmune response is unknown, but it is believed to involve a combination of genetic and environmental factors, such as viral infections.

Because individuals with Type 1 diabetes cannot produce insulin, they must rely on external insulin sources (through injections or an insulin pump) to regulate their blood glucose levels. Managing Type 1 diabetes requires lifelong commitment, including careful monitoring of blood sugar levels, insulin administration, diet, exercise, and regular healthcare checkups.

Type 2 Diabetes (T2D)

Type 2 diabetes is the most common form of the disease, accounting for approximately 90-95% of all diabetes cases worldwide. Unlike Type 1 diabetes, Type 2 diabetes is characterized by insulin resistance, meaning that the body's cells become less responsive to insulin over time. Initially, the pancreas compensates for this resistance by producing more insulin. However, as the disease progresses, the pancreas may struggle to keep up with the demand, and blood sugar levels rise.

Type 2 diabetes is often linked to lifestyle factors, such as being overweight, physically inactive, or having an unhealthy diet. It is most commonly diagnosed in adults, but with the increasing rates of childhood obesity, more young people are being diagnosed with Type 2 diabetes. While insulin is sometimes required for people with Type 2 diabetes, the condition is often managed with lifestyle changes, oral medications, and, in some cases, insulin therapy.

Gestational Diabetes (GDM)

Gestational diabetes occurs during pregnancy and affects about 2-10% of pregnant women, typically developing in the second or third trimester. Like Type 2 diabetes, gestational diabetes is characterized by insulin resistance. During pregnancy, the body produces hormones that can interfere with insulin function, leading to elevated blood sugar levels. While gestational diabetes usually resolves after childbirth, women who experience it are at an increased risk of developing Type 2 diabetes later in life.

Gestational diabetes can also increase the risk of complications during pregnancy, including preeclampsia, premature birth, and an increased likelihood of the baby developing obesity or Type 2 diabetes later in life. Managing gestational diabetes requires careful monitoring of blood glucose levels, dietary changes, and, in some cases, medication.

Latent Autoimmune Diabetes in Adults (LADA)

LADA, sometimes referred to as Type 1.5 diabetes, is a form of autoimmune diabetes that shares features with both Type 1 and Type 2 diabetes. It typically develops in adults over the age of 30 and is often misdiagnosed as Type 2 diabetes due to its slow progression. Like Type 1 diabetes, LADA involves an autoimmune attack on the insulin-producing beta cells of the pancreas, but it usually progresses more slowly. Insulin production may still be present for several years after diagnosis, but eventually, individuals with LADA may need insulin therapy to manage blood glucose levels.

Maturity-Onset Diabetes of the Young (MODY)

MODY is a rare form of diabetes caused by a mutation in a single gene. It is typically diagnosed in adolescents or young adults and is often mistaken for Type 1 or Type 2 diabetes. Unlike Type 1 diabetes, where the immune system destroys insulin-producing cells, MODY involves a genetic defect that leads to insufficient insulin production. Because MODY is genetic, it runs in families, and individuals with MODY may have a family history of early-onset diabetes. Treatment varies depending on the specific genetic mutation, but it often involves lifestyle changes and, in some cases, oral medications.

How the Body Processes Sugar (Glucose)

To understand diabetes more deeply, it is essential to know how glucose is processed in the body under normal circumstances. After we eat, our digestive system breaks down carbohydrates into glucose, which is then absorbed into the bloodstream. This causes a rise in blood sugar levels. In response to the increase in blood sugar, the pancreas releases insulin, which helps transport glucose into cells, where it is either used for energy or stored for later use in the liver and muscles.

Insulin acts like a key, unlocking the door to cells so glucose can enter. Once inside the cells, glucose is either immediately used for energy or stored in the form of glycogen for future use. Insulin also helps regulate blood sugar levels by facilitating the storage of excess glucose in the liver. The liver acts as a glucose reservoir, releasing glucose into the bloodstream when blood sugar levels are low, such as between meals or during physical activity.

In individuals without diabetes, this system of glucose regulation works seamlessly, ensuring blood sugar levels remain within a narrow range, typically between 70-100 mg/dL when fasting. However, in individuals with diabetes, either the insulin production is insufficient (as in Type 1 diabetes) or the body's cells do not respond to insulin effectively (as in Type 2 diabetes), causing blood sugar levels to rise uncontrollably.

Common Misconceptions and Myths About Diabetes

Despite the growing awareness of diabetes, there are still many misconceptions and myths surrounding the disease. These myths can perpetuate misunderstanding and stigma, making it harder for individuals to seek proper care or fully understand their condition.

Myth 1: Diabetes is Caused by Eating Too Much Sugar

One of the most common misconceptions about diabetes is that it is caused by consuming too much sugar. While excessive sugar consumption can contribute to weight gain and insulin resistance, diabetes is not directly caused by eating sugary foods. Type 1 diabetes is an autoimmune disease, while Type 2 diabetes is influenced by genetic factors and lifestyle choices, including diet, exercise, and weight management. Moderation in sugar intake is important, but diabetes is not a consequence of occasional sweet treats.

Myth 2: Only Overweight People Get Type 2 Diabetes

Although being overweight or obese is a significant risk factor for Type 2 diabetes, it is not the sole cause. Many people with Type 2 diabetes are of normal weight or only slightly overweight. Genetics, age, and other environmental factors also play a crucial role in the development of Type 2 diabetes. It's important to recognize that anyone, regardless of body weight, can develop Type 2 diabetes.

Myth 3: People with Diabetes Cannot Eat Carbohydrates

Carbohydrates are often vilified in the context of diabetes management, but they are not inherently bad. In fact, carbohydrates are the body's primary energy source. What matters is the type and amount of carbohydrates consumed. Complex carbohydrates found in whole grains, fruits, and vegetables are digested more slowly and have a less dramatic impact on blood sugar levels compared to simple carbohydrates found in sugary snacks and refined foods. People with diabetes can include carbohydrates in their diet as long as they are mindful of portion sizes and the types of carbs they consume.

Myth 4: Diabetes Is Only a Problem for Older Adults

While Type 2 diabetes is more common in older adults, the disease can affect individuals of all ages. The rise in childhood obesity has led to an increase in Type 2 diabetes diagnoses among children and adolescents. Type 1 diabetes, which is an autoimmune condition, often develops in childhood or adolescence. It is important to understand that diabetes is not confined to any one age group.

Conclusion

Diabetes is a multifaceted condition that affects millions of people around the world. Understanding the science behind the disease, the various types, and the way the body processes glucose is essential for both individuals living with diabetes and those seeking to prevent it. By dispelling myths and misconceptions, we can begin to change the way we view and manage diabetes, empowering people to take control of their health and make informed decisions about their care.

Chapter 2: The Science Behind Diabetes

To truly understand diabetes, it is crucial to dive deeper into the biological processes that underpin the condition. At its core, diabetes is a disruption in the body's ability to regulate blood glucose (sugar) levels, and this disruption is tied to the delicate interplay between insulin, glucose metabolism, and various organs involved in maintaining energy balance. This chapter will explore the role of insulin, how glucose is processed in the body, and the physiological differences between the various types of diabetes. By understanding these mechanisms, we can gain a better appreciation of how the body's natural systems fail in diabetes and how they can be managed or restored.

The Role of Insulin and Glucose Metabolism

Insulin: The Key to Energy Metabolism

Insulin is a hormone produced by the pancreas; a gland located behind the stomach. Its primary function is to regulate the level of glucose in the blood by facilitating the uptake of glucose into cells. Every time we eat, particularly foods rich in carbohydrates, glucose from the digestive system enters the bloodstream. In a healthy individual, this surge in blood sugar triggers the pancreas to release insulin, which acts as a key, allowing glucose to enter cells in tissues such as the liver, muscles, and fat.

Once inside the cells, glucose can either be used immediately for energy or stored for later use. The liver and muscles store glucose in the form of glycogen, a complex carbohydrate that can be converted back into glucose when the body needs energy, such as between meals or during physical activity. Insulin also helps the body store excess glucose in the liver as glycogen and prevents the liver from releasing too much glucose into the bloodstream when it is not needed.

Insulin not only facilitates the uptake of glucose but also plays a role in the metabolism of fat and protein. When glucose is abundant, insulin encourages fat storage by promoting the synthesis of triglycerides in fat cells. It also inhibits the breakdown of fat for energy. In the case of protein, insulin promotes the uptake of amino acids into cells, facilitating the creation of new proteins for muscle growth and repair.

Glucose Homeostasis: Maintaining Blood Sugar Levels

The body operates within a tightly regulated range of blood glucose levels, known as *glucose homeostasis*. This is crucial because both hyperglycemia (high blood sugar) and hypoglycemia (low blood sugar) can be harmful to the body. Under normal conditions, the blood sugar level fluctuates between 70 and 100 mg/dL when fasting. After meals, blood sugar may rise temporarily but should return to baseline levels once insulin takes effect.

Several hormones, including glucagon and cortisol, also play important roles in maintaining glucose balance. When blood sugar levels drop too low, the pancreas releases glucagon, which signals the liver to convert stored glycogen back into glucose and release it into the bloodstream. This process, known as *gluconeogenesis*, ensures the body has enough glucose for essential functions, especially in times of fasting or between meals.

However, when insulin production is insufficient or when the body becomes resistant to insulin, glucose homeostasis is disrupted. This is what leads to the elevated blood sugar levels characteristic of diabetes.

The Physiological Differences Between Types of Diabetes

The most common types of diabetes—Type 1, Type 2, and gestational diabetes—affect the insulin-glucose system in distinct ways. Let's examine the physiological differences that define each form of diabetes.

Type 1 Diabetes: Autoimmune Destruction of Insulin-Producing Cells

In Type 1 diabetes (T1D), the body's immune system mistakenly attacks and destroys the beta cells in the pancreas, which are responsible for producing insulin. This autoimmune response leaves individuals with little to no insulin production. As a result, glucose from the bloodstream cannot enter the cells, and blood glucose levels rise uncontrollably.

Type 1 diabetes is typically diagnosed in children, adolescents, or young adults, but it can occur at any age. Unlike Type 2 diabetes, which is linked to insulin resistance, Type 1 diabetes is primarily a problem of insulin deficiency. Since the pancreas can no longer produce insulin, individuals with Type 1 diabetes must rely on external sources of insulin, which are typically administered through injections or an insulin pump.

In addition to insulin therapy, people with Type 1 diabetes need to carefully monitor their blood glucose levels throughout the day, adjusting insulin doses as needed based on factors such as food intake, physical activity, and stress. Since the body's ability to regulate glucose is compromised, managing Type 1 diabetes involves continuous vigilance and lifestyle modifications.

Physiological Characteristics of Type 1 Diabetes:

- **Cause:** Autoimmune destruction of pancreatic beta cells.
- **Insulin production:** Little to no insulin is produced by the pancreas.
- **Blood glucose levels:** Persistently elevated due to lack of insulin.

- **Management:** Requires lifelong insulin therapy, blood sugar monitoring, diet, and lifestyle management.

Type 2 Diabetes: Insulin Resistance and Impaired Insulin Secretion

Type 2 diabetes (T2D) is the most common form of diabetes, affecting millions of people worldwide. Unlike Type 1 diabetes, where the pancreas cannot produce insulin, Type 2 diabetes is characterized by two key problems: insulin resistance and inadequate insulin production.

Insulin resistance occurs when the body's cells—particularly muscle, fat, and liver cells—become less responsive to insulin. As a result, glucose does not enter cells efficiently, leading to elevated blood glucose levels. In response to this resistance, the pancreas produces more insulin in an attempt to compensate for the reduced effectiveness of the hormone. Over time, however, the pancreas becomes unable to keep up with the increased demand, and insulin production may decrease.

The primary risk factors for Type 2 diabetes include obesity, physical inactivity, poor diet, genetics, and aging. Although Type 2 diabetes was once considered an adult-onset disease, it is increasingly being diagnosed in children and adolescents, particularly in those who are overweight or obese.

The management of Type 2 diabetes often involves lifestyle changes, such as adopting a healthier diet, increasing physical activity, and losing weight. Many people with Type 2 diabetes also require oral medications, such as metformin, or even insulin injections to manage their blood sugar levels.

Physiological Characteristics of Type 2 Diabetes

- **Cause:** Insulin resistance and eventual pancreatic beta cell dysfunction.

- **Insulin production:** Initially, insulin production is high, but the pancreas becomes less able to produce enough insulin over time.
- **Blood glucose levels:** Elevated due to insulin resistance and impaired insulin secretion.
- **Management:** Lifestyle changes (diet and exercise), oral medications, and sometimes insulin therapy.

Gestational Diabetes: Temporary Insulin Resistance During Pregnancy

Gestational diabetes is a form of diabetes that occurs during pregnancy, typically in the second or third trimester. It is characterized by insulin resistance, which develops as a result of hormonal changes during pregnancy. The placenta produces hormones that can interfere with insulin's ability to help glucose enter the cells, leading to elevated blood glucose levels.

Although gestational diabetes usually resolves after childbirth, it can increase the risk of complications for both the mother and the baby. Women who develop gestational diabetes are at a higher risk of developing Type 2 diabetes later in life, and their children may also be at a greater risk of obesity and Type 2 diabetes as they grow older. Gestational diabetes is typically diagnosed through blood glucose testing during pregnancy, and it is managed through careful monitoring of blood sugar levels, dietary modifications, and, in some cases, insulin therapy.

Physiological Characteristics of Gestational Diabetes

- **Cause:** Insulin resistance caused by pregnancy-related hormonal changes.
- **Insulin production:** Initially sufficient, but the body's ability to utilize insulin is impaired during pregnancy.

- **Blood glucose levels:** Elevated during pregnancy due to insulin resistance.
- **Management:** Diet, exercise, blood glucose monitoring, and possibly insulin therapy during pregnancy.

LADA (Latent Autoimmune Diabetes in Adults): A Hybrid Between Type 1 and Type 2 Diabetes

LADA, also known as Type 1.5 diabetes, is a form of autoimmune diabetes that shares features of both Type 1 and Type 2 diabetes. It typically develops in adults, usually after the age of 30, and is often misdiagnosed as Type 2 diabetes because it progresses slowly. In LADA, the immune system begins to attack the insulin-producing beta cells of the pancreas, much like in Type 1 diabetes. However, the autoimmune attack is less aggressive and occurs over a longer period, meaning insulin production can remain relatively high for some time before it declines.

The hallmark of LADA is that individuals initially do not require insulin therapy, but as the disease progresses, insulin production becomes insufficient, and external insulin therapy may eventually be necessary.

Physiological Characteristics of LADA

- **Cause:** Autoimmune destruction of pancreatic beta cells (like Type 1).
- **Insulin production:** Initially normal but decreases over time as beta cells are destroyed.
- **Blood glucose levels:** Initially elevated, but typically manage with oral medications before requiring insulin.
- **Management:** Lifestyle changes, oral medications, and eventually insulin therapy as the disease progresses.

Conclusion

The science behind diabetes is intricate, involving a complex network of hormones, cells, and organs working together to regulate glucose metabolism. At the heart of the condition is insulin, a vital hormone that facilitates the uptake of glucose into cells for energy. When this system is disrupted, whether through autoimmune destruction of insulin-producing cells (Type 1), insulin resistance (Type 2), or pregnancy-related changes (gestational diabetes), blood glucose levels become abnormally high, leading to the hallmark symptoms and long-term complications of diabetes.

Understanding the physiological mechanisms of diabetes not only sheds light on why the disease develops in the first place, but it also provides insight into the different types of diabetes and how they affect the body. With this knowledge, individuals living with diabetes can make informed decisions about their care, helping to manage the disease and improve quality of life.

Chapter 3

Insulin Resistance and Beta Cells

One of the most fundamental mechanisms that underpins many forms of diabetes—especially Type 2 and gestational diabetes—is **insulin resistance**, a condition where the body's cells become less responsive to insulin. This chapter explores the development of insulin resistance, the critical role of beta cells in regulating blood glucose, and the pathophysiology of insulin resistance in Type 2 and gestational diabetes. By understanding how insulin resistance develops and how beta cells attempt to compensate for it, we can gain insight into the underlying causes of these forms of diabetes and how they affect the body.

The Role of Beta Cells and Insulin in Blood Sugar Regulation

To appreciate how insulin resistance develops, it is essential to first understand the role of insulin and the function of the pancreas, specifically the **beta cells**.

Insulin is a hormone produced and secreted by **beta cells**, which are located in the **islets of Langerhans** in the pancreas. Its main function is to regulate blood glucose levels by promoting the uptake of glucose into cells, particularly muscle, liver, and fat cells. When glucose from food enters the bloodstream after digestion, it triggers the pancreas to release insulin. Insulin acts as a key that allows glucose to enter these cells, where it is either used immediately for energy or stored for later use.

- **Liver cells** store glucose in the form of glycogen.
- **Muscle cells** use glucose for energy or store it as glycogen.
- **Fat cells** store glucose as fat, which can later be used for energy.

Under normal conditions, the pancreas releases just the right amount of insulin to maintain blood glucose levels within a narrow, healthy range—typically between 70 and 100 mg/dL when fasting. When blood sugar levels rise (such as after eating), insulin facilitates the uptake of glucose by cells, helping to bring blood sugar levels back down to normal.

In individuals with **insulin resistance**, however, the body's cells do not respond to insulin as effectively. This causes glucose to remain in the bloodstream instead of being absorbed into cells, leading to **elevated blood glucose levels**. In response, the pancreas works harder to produce more insulin to overcome the resistance. For a time, this compensatory mechanism may keep blood sugar levels relatively stable, but over time, the pancreas becomes unable to produce enough insulin to meet the body's needs, contributing to the development of **hyperglycemia** (high blood sugar).

How Insulin Resistance Develops

Insulin resistance is the result of complex interactions between genetic factors, lifestyle choices, and environmental influences. The exact cause of insulin resistance is not fully understood, but several factors have been identified as contributing to its development:

Obesity and Excess Fat Tissue

One of the most significant risk factors for insulin resistance is **obesity**, particularly **visceral fat**—fat stored deep in the abdominal area that surrounds vital organs like the liver and pancreas. Fat cells, especially those in the abdominal region, are metabolically active and secrete various substances known as **adipokines**. Some adipokines, such as **Resistin** and **TNF-alpha**, promote inflammation and interfere with the action of insulin, making it harder for insulin to effectively transport glucose into cells.

In addition, excess fat accumulation leads to increased levels of **free fatty acids** in the bloodstream. Elevated free fatty acids can also impair the ability of muscle cells to take up glucose, exacerbating insulin resistance.

Physical Inactivity

A sedentary lifestyle is another major contributor to insulin resistance. Regular physical activity helps improve the efficiency of insulin by increasing the number of insulin receptors on muscle cells and enhancing their ability to take up glucose. Conversely, a lack of physical activity reduces this insulin sensitivity. In people who are inactive, the body's cells become less responsive to insulin, leading to higher blood glucose levels.

Poor Diet

Dietary habits play a critical role in the development of insulin resistance. Diets high in **refined carbohydrates**, **sugars**, and **saturated fats** can contribute to insulin resistance. These foods cause rapid spikes in blood sugar and insulin levels, and over time, this can lead to **insulin overproduction**. Chronic overproduction of insulin can strain the beta cells in the pancreas, eventually leading to beta cell dysfunction.

Conversely, **fiber-rich diets** that include whole grains, vegetables, and legumes, as well as **healthy fats** (such as those found in olive oil and avocados), have been shown to improve insulin sensitivity and reduce the risk of developing insulin resistance.

Genetic Factors

Genetics also play a role in determining who is more susceptible to insulin resistance. Family history is a strong predictor of risk for insulin resistance and Type 2 diabetes. Specific genes related to insulin signaling pathways, fat storage, and glucose metabolism may influence an individual's likelihood of developing insulin resistance. However, environmental factors such as diet, physical activity, and weight can modify the impact of genetic predisposition.

Aging

As people age, their insulin sensitivity naturally declines. This means that older adults are more likely to develop insulin resistance. Aging also often correlates with weight gain, especially around the abdomen, which can further contribute to insulin resistance. Additionally, a decrease in physical activity and muscle mass in older adults can reduce insulin sensitivity, making blood sugar regulation more difficult.

Insulin Resistance in Type 2 Diabetes

In **Type 2 diabetes (T2D)**, the development of insulin resistance is the central pathological feature. Type 2 diabetes is primarily a disease of **insulin resistance**, in which the body's cells (especially muscle and fat cells) do not respond to insulin properly. Initially, the pancreas compensates for this resistance by producing more insulin. As insulin production increases, the pancreas can often maintain relatively normal blood glucose levels.

However, over time, the pancreas becomes unable to produce enough insulin to overcome the resistance. This leads to chronic **hyperglycemia** (high blood sugar), which, if left untreated, can result in complications affecting the heart, kidneys, eyes, and nerves. The progression of insulin resistance in Type 2 diabetes typically follows a slow and insidious course, with symptoms often developing gradually over many years before a formal diagnosis is made.

The pathophysiology of insulin resistance in Type 2 diabetes involves multiple metabolic disturbances:

1. **Impaired Insulin Signaling:** Insulin resistance begins with a breakdown in insulin signaling. Normally, when insulin binds to its receptor on a cell's surface, it triggers a cascade of signals that allows glucose to enter the cell. In insulin-resistant individuals, this signaling pathway is disrupted, preventing glucose uptake.

2. **Increased Glucose Production by the Liver:** The liver plays an essential role in maintaining glucose balance by storing glucose as glycogen and releasing it as needed. In insulin resistance, the liver becomes less responsive to insulin and continues to produce glucose (via gluconeogenesis) even when blood sugar levels are high, exacerbating hyperglycemia.

3. **Beta Cell Dysfunction:** Over time, the pancreas' beta cells become overworked due to the increased demand for insulin. Initially, they compensate by producing more insulin, but as beta cell function declines, insulin secretion becomes insufficient to manage blood glucose levels, leading to the onset of Type 2 diabetes.

Insulin Resistance in Gestational Diabetes

Gestational diabetes occurs during pregnancy, typically in the second or third trimester, and is characterized by **insulin resistance** combined with insufficient insulin production. During pregnancy, the placenta releases hormones (such as human placental lactogen, cortisol, and estrogen) that can make the body less responsive to insulin. This creates a condition of **physiological insulin resistance**, meaning that the body requires more insulin to maintain normal blood glucose levels. In a healthy pregnancy, the pancreas is usually able to produce enough additional insulin to compensate for this resistance. However, in some women, especially those who are overweight, have a family history of diabetes, or are carrying multiples, the pancreas cannot produce enough insulin to meet the increased demands, leading to **gestational diabetes**.

Gestational diabetes can have significant consequences for both mother and baby. Elevated blood glucose levels during pregnancy can lead to **macrosomia**, a condition where the baby grows too large, increasing the risk of complications during childbirth. Gestational diabetes also increases the risk of **pre-eclampsia**, a dangerous rise in blood pressure during pregnancy.

Gestational diabetes typically resolves after childbirth, but women who experience it are at a higher risk of developing **Type 2 diabetes** later in life. Babies born to mothers with gestational diabetes are also more likely to become overweight and develop Type 2 diabetes as they grow older.

Conclusion

Insulin resistance is a central mechanism in many forms of diabetes, particularly **Type 2** and **gestational diabetes**. Insulin resistance occurs when the body's cells fail to respond properly to insulin, leading to elevated blood glucose levels. In Type 2 diabetes, insulin resistance is compounded by beta cell dysfunction, where the pancreas is unable to produce enough insulin to keep blood glucose levels in check. In gestational diabetes, insulin resistance develops due to hormonal changes during pregnancy, leading to temporary glucose intolerance.

The pathophysiology of insulin resistance is influenced by a combination of genetic, environmental, and lifestyle factors. Understanding the underlying mechanisms that cause insulin resistance is essential for managing and preventing the progression of diabetes. Through dietary modifications, regular physical activity, weight management, and medication, individuals can improve insulin sensitivity, manage blood sugar levels, and reduce the risk of complications associated with diabetes.

In the next chapters, we will explore in more detail how insulin resistance is diagnosed, how lifestyle changes can help improve insulin sensitivity, and what treatments are available to manage blood sugar levels effectively.

Chapter 4

Blood Sugar Regulation and Homeostasis

Blood sugar regulation is one of the most critical processes in the human body. Maintaining balanced glucose levels is essential not only for energy production but also for the proper functioning of organs and tissues. When the body's mechanisms of blood sugar regulation go awry, as is the case in diabetes, it can lead to a cascade of health problems, ranging from fatigue and nerve damage to heart disease and kidney failure. In this chapter, we will explore the intricate processes involved in blood sugar regulation, how they become disrupted in diabetes, and the importance of maintaining a healthy balance. We will also discuss how to interpret blood sugar readings and how they guide the management of diabetes.

What Is Blood Sugar Regulation?

Blood sugar, or **glucose**, is the body's primary source of energy. It fuels cells, tissues, and organs, especially the brain, which relies almost exclusively on glucose for its functions. Maintaining blood glucose within a narrow, healthy range is crucial for the body to function optimally. This balance is achieved through a complex system of hormonal regulation, primarily involving **insulin** and **glucagon**, as well as several other hormones that help maintain glucose homeostasis.

The body has evolved several mechanisms to ensure that blood glucose levels remain stable, despite fluctuations caused by food intake, physical activity, and periods of fasting. These mechanisms involve multiple organs, including the **pancreas, liver, muscles**, and **adipose tissue** (fat cells), all of which interact in a finely tuned feedback loop.

Key Hormones Involved in Blood Sugar Regulation

Insulin: The Blood Sugar Regulator

The pancreas plays a central role in blood sugar regulation, and **insulin**, produced by **beta cells** in the pancreas, is the body's primary hormone for lowering blood sugar. After eating, glucose from food enters the bloodstream, and the rise in blood sugar signals the pancreas to release insulin. Insulin acts like a key, enabling glucose to enter cells for energy or storage. It facilitates glucose uptake by muscle and fat cells, where it can be used for immediate energy or stored as glycogen in the liver and muscles for later use.

- **In the liver**, insulin promotes the storage of glucose as glycogen, reducing the amount of glucose circulating in the bloodstream.

- **In muscles and fat tissue**, insulin facilitates the uptake of glucose to be used as fuel or stored for future energy needs.

Glucagon: The Counterbalance to Insulin

While insulin is responsible for lowering blood glucose levels, **glucagon**, another hormone secreted by the pancreas, works to raise blood sugar levels when they are too low. When blood glucose levels fall (such as between meals or during exercise), the pancreas releases glucagon into the bloodstream.

Glucagon signals the liver to break down glycogen into glucose and release it into the bloodstream, a process known as **glycogenolysis**. If glucose stores in the liver are depleted, glucagon also stimulates the liver to produce new glucose through a process called **gluconeogenesis**.

This delicate balance between insulin and glucagon ensures that blood glucose levels do not drop too low (hypoglycemia) or rise too high (hyperglycemia).

Other Hormones That Influence Blood Sugar

In addition to insulin and glucagon, several other hormones play a role in blood sugar regulation:

- **Cortisol**, often called the "stress hormone," can increase blood glucose levels. It is released during times of stress and helps ensure that the body has enough energy to respond to the stressor by promoting the breakdown of proteins and fats into glucose.

- **Epinephrine (adrenaline)**, also released during stress, can stimulate the liver to release glucose and increase blood flow to muscles, preparing the body for the "fight-or-flight" response.

- **Growth hormone** helps regulate glucose metabolism and can increase blood glucose levels by inhibiting the action of insulin.

Together, these hormones create a complex system that helps the body adapt to various conditions, ensuring that energy needs are met while avoiding dangerous fluctuations in blood sugar levels.

How Blood Sugar Regulation Goes Awry in Diabetes

In individuals with **diabetes**, the body's ability to regulate blood sugar is impaired. The mechanisms that normally work in harmony to maintain blood sugar homeostasis fail, leading to chronic hyperglycemia (high blood sugar), which can cause significant damage to organs and tissues over time. The disruptions in blood sugar regulation differ between the various types of diabetes, but in all cases, the result is an inability to maintain balanced blood glucose levels.

Type 1 Diabetes: Lack of Insulin Production

In **Type 1 diabetes (T1D)**, the immune system mistakenly attacks and destroys the beta cells in the pancreas, leading to a complete lack of insulin production. Without insulin, glucose cannot enter cells, and it builds up in the bloodstream. The body attempts to compensate for the lack of insulin by breaking down fat for energy, leading to weight loss and an increase in ketones, which can lead to a dangerous condition known as **diabetic ketoacidosis (DKA)**. Because the pancreas cannot produce insulin in Type 1 diabetes, individuals must rely on external insulin through injections or an insulin pump to regulate their blood sugar.

Type 2 Diabetes: Insulin Resistance and Beta Cell Dysfunction

In **Type 2 diabetes (T2D)**, the problem begins with **insulin resistance**. The cells in the body, particularly in the liver, muscles, and fat tissue, become less responsive to insulin, meaning they do not take up glucose efficiently. In response, the pancreas produces more insulin to overcome the resistance, but over time, the beta cells become exhausted and can no longer produce enough insulin to meet the body's needs. This results in elevated blood glucose levels.

As the condition progresses, the liver may also continue to produce glucose, despite the presence of high blood sugar, exacerbating hyperglycemia. Insulin resistance, combined with a decline in insulin production, causes the blood sugar to become increasingly difficult to control.

Gestational Diabetes: Hormonal Insulin Resistance During Pregnancy

Gestational diabetes occurs during pregnancy when the body becomes less responsive to insulin, typically due to hormonal changes. As pregnancy progresses, the placenta releases hormones such as **human placental lactogen** (HPL), **cortisol**, and **progesterone**, which can make the body more insulin resistant. The pancreas tries to compensate by producing more insulin, but in some women, the pancreas cannot keep up with the increased demand, leading to elevated blood sugar levels. Although gestational diabetes usually resolves after childbirth, it increases the risk of developing Type 2 diabetes later in life.

The Importance of Maintaining Blood Sugar Balance

Maintaining blood sugar balance is crucial for both short-term and long-term health. When blood sugar levels are too high (hyperglycemia), it can damage blood vessels, nerves, and organs over time. Chronic high blood sugar is a major contributor to the long-term complications of diabetes, including:

- **Cardiovascular disease**, as high blood sugar can damage blood vessels, increasing the risk of heart attacks and strokes.
- **Kidney damage (diabetic nephropathy)**, which can lead to kidney failure.
- **Nerve damage (diabetic neuropathy)**, which can result in numbness, tingling, and pain, especially in the extremities.
- **Vision problems**, including diabetic retinopathy, which can lead to blindness.
- **Poor wound healing** and increased susceptibility to infections.

On the other hand, when blood sugar levels are too low (hypoglycemia), it can cause immediate symptoms such as dizziness, confusion, and even loss of consciousness. Severe hypoglycemia can be life-threatening if not treated promptly.

Achieving balance in blood sugar is essential to preventing both immediate and long-term complications. This requires careful monitoring of blood glucose levels, making lifestyle changes, and in some cases, taking medication or insulin to ensure that blood sugar remains within the target range.

Understanding Blood Sugar Readings

Blood glucose levels are typically measured through blood tests, and the readings provide critical information for managing diabetes. It is important to understand how to interpret these readings and what they mean for blood sugar control.

1. Normal Blood Sugar Levels

- **Fasting blood glucose (before meals):** 70–100 mg/dL.
- **Post-meal (2 hours after eating):** Less than 140 mg/dL.
- **Hemoglobin A1c (average blood sugar over 2-3 months):** Below 5.7%.

2. Prediabetes

- **Fasting blood glucose:** 100–125 mg/dL.
- **Post-meal:** 140–199 mg/dL.
- **A1c:** 5.7–6.4%.

3. Diabetes

- **Fasting blood glucose:** 126 mg/dL or higher.
- **Post-meal:** 200 mg/dL or higher.
- **A1c:** 6.5% or higher.

Hypoglycemia

Blood glucose below 70 mg/dL is considered low and may require immediate intervention, such as consuming fast-acting carbohydrates (e.g., glucose tablets, juice).

By regularly monitoring blood sugar levels, people with diabetes can adjust their diet, exercise, and medication to keep blood sugar within the target range and reduce the risk of complications.

Conclusion

Blood sugar regulation is a highly complex, dynamic process that is essential for overall health. Insulin, glucagon, and other hormones work together to ensure that glucose levels stay within a healthy range, adapting to various factors such as food intake, exercise, and stress. When these systems fail, as in diabetes, it can lead to chronic hyperglycemia and a range of health complications.

Understanding how blood sugar regulation works and how it can become disrupted in diabetes is critical for managing the disease. By monitoring blood glucose levels, making lifestyle changes, and using appropriate medications, individuals with diabetes can achieve better blood sugar control and improve their quality of life.

Chapter 5

Understanding HbA1c: A Key to Blood Sugar Control

When it comes to managing diabetes, one of the most valuable indicators of long-term blood sugar control is the **Hemoglobin A1c (HbA1c) test**. This test provides a snapshot of your average blood glucose levels over the past two to three months, offering important insights into how well your diabetes is being managed. Unlike daily blood glucose monitoring, which can fluctuate throughout the day depending on various factors, HbA1c provides a more consistent and long-term view of blood sugar regulation. In this chapter, we will explore what HbA1c is, how it reflects blood sugar control, how it is used in diagnosis and treatment decisions, and why maintaining an optimal HbA1c level is crucial for overall health.

What is HbA1c?

To understand the significance of the HbA1c test, it's important to first know what **HbA1c** refers to. Hemoglobin is a protein found in red blood cells that binds to oxygen and carries it throughout the body. Each red blood cell has a lifespan of about **120 days**, and over that period, it can interact with glucose in the bloodstream. When glucose enters the bloodstream, it can attach to hemoglobin in a process known as **glycation**.

The more glucose present in the blood, the higher the amount of glycated hemoglobin (HbA1c). Essentially, HbA1c is a measure of the percentage of hemoglobin in your red blood cells that has glucose attached to it. The higher your average blood sugar levels over the past few months, the higher your HbA1c will be.

The advantage of the HbA1c test is that it reflects the average blood sugar levels over a long period, unlike a fasting blood glucose test or a post-meal glucose test, which provide a snapshot of blood sugar at a specific point in time. This makes HbA1c an excellent tool for evaluating long-term blood sugar control, providing both patients and healthcare providers with a clear picture of how well diabetes is being managed.

Why is HbA1c Important for Diabetes Management?

The **HbA1c test** is considered a **gold standard** for monitoring and managing diabetes for several reasons:

1. **Reflects Long-Term Blood Sugar Control:** The HbA1c test shows the average level of glucose in the blood over a period of **2 to 3 months**, which corresponds to the lifespan of red blood cells. This is important because it gives healthcare providers a clear picture of how well someone's blood sugar has been controlled over time, rather than being influenced by the fluctuations that can happen during a single day. For individuals with diabetes, maintaining consistent blood glucose levels is crucial to reducing the risk of complications.

2. **Indicates Risk of Complications:** Elevated HbA1c levels are associated with an increased risk of developing complications from diabetes, such as **cardiovascular disease, kidney damage, nerve damage**, and **vision problems**. By regularly monitoring HbA1c levels, healthcare providers can assess whether blood glucose control is adequate and make adjustments to treatment plans as needed.

3. **Guides Treatment Adjustments:** HbA1c provides valuable feedback on how well an individual's diabetes management plan is working. If HbA1c levels are too high, it signals that blood sugar levels have been consistently high over the past few months, and adjustments to treatment—such as medication, diet, exercise, or insulin therapy—may be necessary. Conversely, if HbA1c levels are within the target range, it indicates that the current management plan is effective.

How is HbA1c Measured?

The HbA1c test is typically performed using a blood sample, which can be taken from a vein in your arm or with a fingerstick. The laboratory then analyzes the blood sample and provides an **HbA1c percentage** result.

An HbA1c result is expressed as a percentage, which reflects the amount of glycated hemoglobin in the blood:

- **Normal HbA1c:** Less than 5.7%
- **Prediabetes (impaired glucose tolerance):** 5.7% to 6.4%
- **Diabetes:** 6.5% or higher

  In people without diabetes, the typical HbA1c is **below 5.7%**, meaning that their average blood glucose levels remain in the normal range. For those with **prediabetes**, an HbA1c between **5.7% and 6.4%** indicates a higher risk of developing Type 2 diabetes if lifestyle changes are not made. An HbA1c of **6.5% or higher** is used for the diagnosis of **diabetes**.

Target HbA1c Levels for People with Diabetes

For people diagnosed with diabetes, the goal is to maintain an HbA1c level as close to normal as possible, typically below **7%**. However, individual targets may vary depending on several factors, including age, overall health, and the presence of any diabetes-related complications. Here's a general guideline for target HbA1c levels:

- **For most adults with diabetes**: The general target is **less than 7%**. This level has been shown to reduce the risk of long-term complications associated with high blood sugar.

- **For older adults, those with multiple health conditions, or those at risk of hypoglycemia**: A less stringent target, such as **7.5% to 8%**, may be appropriate, as tight control could increase the risk of low blood sugar (hypoglycemia) in these individuals.

- **For children or young adults with Type 1 diabetes**: The target might be closer to **7%** or lower, depending on the specific circumstances.

How HbA1c Levels Guide Diagnosis and Treatment

1. **Diagnosis of Diabetes and Prediabetes:** HbA1c is a key tool for diagnosing both diabetes and prediabetes. For diagnosis:
   - **HbA1c of 6.5% or higher** is considered diagnostic for diabetes.
   - **HbA1c between 5.7% and 6.4%** indicates prediabetes, which signals the need for lifestyle changes to prevent or delay the onset of Type 2 diabetes.

   The **American Diabetes Association (ADA)** and other health organizations recommend HbA1c testing as part of routine screening for diabetes, especially for individuals at higher risk (e.g., those with a family history of diabetes, obesity, or older age).

2. **Guiding Treatment Decisions:** HbA1c levels play a pivotal role in guiding treatment decisions for people with diabetes:
   - **If HbA1c is above target**: A high HbA1c suggests that blood sugar levels have been consistently high. This could indicate that

the current treatment regimen (medications, insulin, lifestyle changes) is not sufficient, and adjustments may be needed. Possible changes could include adding or adjusting medications, increasing physical activity, or modifying diet.

- o **If HbA1c is at or near target**: This indicates good control of blood sugar. However, it is still important to continue regular monitoring to ensure that the target level is maintained and to detect any potential fluctuations before they become problematic.

3. **Evaluating the Effectiveness of Treatment:** HbA1c is useful in monitoring the effectiveness of treatment strategies. For example:

- o **For Type 1 diabetes**: Regular HbA1c testing helps determine how well the balance between insulin doses, diet, and exercise is maintaining blood glucose levels.
- o **For Type 2 diabetes**: HbA1c serves as a barometer for lifestyle interventions, such as weight loss and exercise, as well as the effectiveness of oral medications or insulin.

Managing HbA1c Levels: Lifestyle and Medication

Achieving and maintaining an optimal HbA1c level involves a combination of lifestyle changes, consistent monitoring, and, when necessary, medication.

1. **Diet and Nutrition**: A balanced diet plays a key role in managing blood sugar levels. Focus on whole, unprocessed foods such as vegetables, lean proteins, whole grains, and healthy fats. Limiting refined sugars and carbohydrates, which can cause blood sugar spikes, is also critical.

2. **Physical Activity**: Regular physical activity helps increase insulin sensitivity, allowing cells to use glucose more effectively. Both aerobic

exercise (such as walking, cycling, swimming) and strength training (such as weight lifting) are beneficial for managing blood sugar.

3. **Medication**: For those with diabetes, medications may be required to help manage blood glucose. This can include **oral medications**, such as **metformin** (which improves insulin sensitivity), or **insulin therapy** for those with Type 1 diabetes or advanced Type 2 diabetes.

4. **Monitoring**: Regular monitoring of blood glucose levels allows individuals to track their daily fluctuations, while HbA1c provides a longer-term view. This combination helps adjust lifestyle and treatment plans as needed.

Understanding the Limitations of HbA1c

While HbA1c is an important and reliable tool for assessing blood sugar control, it does have some limitations:

- **Not suitable for everyone**: Certain conditions, such as **anemia** or **sickle cell disease**, can affect red blood cell turnover, leading to inaccurate HbA1c readings.

- **Variability**: HbA1c levels can vary slightly between individuals due to genetic differences, and they may not fully reflect blood glucose fluctuations, especially in people with very unstable blood sugar. Despite these limitations, HbA1c remains one of the most important tests for managing diabetes and assessing long-term blood sugar control.

Conclusion

HbA1c is a cornerstone of diabetes management, offering a clear and reliable picture of a person's average blood sugar levels over the past few months. It is an essential tool for diagnosing diabetes, setting treatment goals, and monitoring the effectiveness of interventions. Understanding HbA1c and its role in diabetes management is crucial for both people living with diabetes and healthcare providers. By maintaining HbA1c within a healthy range, individuals can significantly reduce their risk of complications and enjoy a better quality of life.

Chapter 6

Type 1 Diabetes – The Autoimmune Condition

Type 1 diabetes (T1D) is a chronic autoimmune condition that occurs when the body's immune system mistakenly attacks and destroys the **insulin-producing beta cells** in the **pancreas**. As a result, individuals with Type 1 diabetes lose the ability to produce insulin, a hormone that plays a critical role in regulating blood sugar (glucose) levels. Unlike Type 2 diabetes, which is often related to insulin resistance and lifestyle factors, Type 1 diabetes is an autoimmune disorder that typically develops in childhood or early adulthood, though it can occur at any age. In this chapter, we will explore how Type 1 diabetes is caused by an autoimmune attack, the symptoms and early warning signs, the process of diagnosis, and the challenges faced by individuals living with the condition.

The Immune System's Role in Type 1 Diabetes

Type 1 diabetes is an **autoimmune disease**, meaning it results from an abnormal response of the body's immune system. Under normal circumstances, the immune system is responsible for defending the body against harmful invaders such as bacteria and viruses. However, in people with Type 1 diabetes, the immune system attacks healthy cells in the body by mistake.

In the case of Type 1 diabetes, the target of this misguided immune response is the **beta cells** of the pancreas. Beta cells are responsible for producing **insulin**, the hormone that helps regulate blood glucose levels by facilitating the uptake of glucose into cells. When the immune system destroys these beta cells, the pancreas is no longer able to produce insulin, resulting in elevated blood glucose levels—a condition known as **hyperglycemia**.

The exact cause of this autoimmune response is not fully understood, but it is believed to be a combination of genetic and environmental factors. Certain genes may predispose individuals to Type 1 diabetes, but environmental triggers, such as viral infections or other unknown factors, are thought to activate the immune system to attack the beta cells.

Genetic Factors in Type 1 Diabetes

While Type 1 diabetes is not directly inherited in the way that some other conditions are, there is a genetic component. Certain genes, particularly those related to the **human leukocyte antigen (HLA) system**, are associated with an increased risk of developing Type 1 diabetes. The HLA system plays a crucial role in immune system function and helps the body distinguish between self and non-self (foreign) cells.

Having a family member with Type 1 diabetes increases the risk of developing the condition, though the majority of people diagnosed with Type 1 diabetes do not have a family history. This suggests that other factors, likely environmental, contribute to the development of the disease.

How Type 1 Diabetes Develops

The development of Type 1 diabetes typically occurs in several stages:

1. **Genetic Predisposition**: Individuals inherit certain genes that make them more susceptible to Type 1 diabetes, although not everyone with these genes will develop the disease.

2. **Immune System Trigger**: An environmental factor, such as a viral infection (e.g., enterovirus, rubella, or cytomegalovirus), may trigger the immune system to mistakenly attack the beta cells in the pancreas.

3. **Beta Cell Destruction**: Over time, the immune system continues to destroy beta cells, leading to a gradual decrease in insulin production.

4. **Insulin Deficiency**: As the beta cells are destroyed, the pancreas produces less and less insulin. Eventually, the body cannot produce enough insulin to regulate blood glucose levels, resulting in high blood sugar and the onset of symptoms.

5. **Onset of Symptoms**: Symptoms often appear suddenly and can be severe. By the time symptoms are noticeable, a significant amount of beta cell function may already be lost.

Symptoms of Type 1 Diabetes

The symptoms of Type 1 diabetes can develop quickly and may include:

- **Excessive Thirst (Polydipsia)**: Due to high blood sugar, the body attempts to get rid of excess glucose through urine, leading to dehydration and a constant feeling of thirst.

- **Frequent Urination (Polyuria)**: As the kidneys work to filter out the excess glucose, this leads to frequent urination. People with Type 1 diabetes may need to urinate several times during the night.

- **Extreme Hunger (Polyphagia)**: Without enough insulin to move glucose into cells, the body's cells cannot access the energy they need. This leads to feelings of hunger, even after eating.

- **Unexplained Weight Loss**: Despite eating more, individuals with Type 1 diabetes may lose weight. This occurs because the body starts breaking down fat and muscle for energy due to the inability to use glucose effectively.

- **Fatigue**: As the body is unable to efficiently utilize glucose, people with Type 1 diabetes often experience persistent tiredness and lack of energy.
- **Blurred Vision**: High blood sugar levels can lead to fluid being pulled from tissues, including the lenses of the eyes, which can cause blurred vision.
- **Nausea and Vomiting**: When the body begins to break down fat for energy, it produces **ketones**—byproducts that can accumulate in the bloodstream, leading to a condition called **diabetic ketoacidosis (DKA)**, which can cause nausea, vomiting, and abdominal pain.

These symptoms often emerge suddenly, and if left untreated, they can lead to serious complications, including **diabetic ketoacidosis (DKA)**, which is a life-threatening condition characterized by very high blood sugar levels and the presence of ketones in the blood.

Early Signs of Type 1 Diabetes

The early signs of Type 1 diabetes can be subtle, but they tend to worsen over time as the pancreas loses more and more beta cells. Parents, caregivers, and individuals should be aware of the following early indicators:

- **Increased thirst and urination**: Children or adults with Type 1 diabetes may begin drinking excessively or needing to urinate more frequently.
- **Tiredness and lethargy**: Persistent tiredness, weakness, or irritability can be an early sign that blood sugar levels are out of balance.
- **Weight loss despite normal or increased eating**: In children, unexplained weight loss, despite a normal appetite or even increased food intake, is a major red flag.

- **Mood swings or irritability**: Fluctuations in blood sugar levels, especially high blood sugar, can cause mood changes and irritability.

- **Fruity-smelling breath**: When the body starts breaking down fat for energy instead of glucose, it produces **ketones**, which can give the breath a fruity or acetone-like smell—a sign of diabetic ketoacidosis (DKA).

Diagnosis of Type 1 Diabetes

The diagnosis of Type 1 diabetes involves several steps, including medical history, physical examination, and laboratory tests. The diagnosis is typically confirmed through the following tests:

1. **Fasting Blood Glucose Test**: This test measures blood sugar levels after an overnight fast. A fasting blood glucose level of **126 mg/dL (7.0 mmol/L) or higher** is indicative of diabetes.

2. **Random Blood Glucose Test**: A blood test taken at any time of the day, regardless of when the person last ate. A random blood glucose level of **200 mg/dL (11.1 mmol/L) or higher**, along with symptoms of diabetes, is suggestive of Type 1 diabetes.

3. **Oral Glucose Tolerance Test (OGTT)**: This test measures how the body responds to a dose of glucose. Although more commonly used in the diagnosis of Type 2 diabetes, it may occasionally be used to evaluate Type 1 diabetes.

4. **Hemoglobin A1c Test**: While the A1c test is commonly used to monitor long-term blood sugar control in people with diagnosed diabetes, it may also be used as a diagnostic tool. An A1c of **6.5% or higher** is a sign of diabetes, but it is not always used in the initial diagnosis of Type 1 diabetes due to the rapid onset of symptoms.

5. **C-Peptide Test**: The C-peptide test measures the amount of insulin produced by the pancreas. In Type 1 diabetes, the C-peptide level is usually low, reflecting the body's inability to produce insulin.

6. **Autoantibody Tests**: People with Type 1 diabetes typically have elevated levels of **autoantibodies** (e.g., **GAD65**, **ICA**, **IA2**), which are markers of autoimmune activity. These tests can help differentiate Type 1 diabetes from other types of diabetes, such as Type 2.

Living with Type 1 Diabetes

Type 1 diabetes is a lifelong condition that requires ongoing management to prevent complications. Because insulin is no longer produced by the body, individuals with Type 1 diabetes must rely on **insulin therapy** to manage their blood glucose levels. Insulin is typically administered through injections or an **insulin pump**, and the dosage must be carefully matched to food intake, physical activity, and blood glucose levels.

Managing Type 1 diabetes also involves regular blood glucose monitoring, ideally using a continuous glucose monitor (CGM) or periodic fingerstick tests. Along with insulin therapy, individuals must focus on maintaining a balanced diet, engaging in regular physical activity, and learning to recognize and manage episodes of low or high blood sugar.

Challenges and Support: The daily demands of managing Type 1 diabetes can be physically and emotionally taxing. People with Type 1 diabetes may face challenges such as the risk of hypoglycemia (low blood sugar) and the constant need to balance insulin intake with food and exercise. Support from healthcare teams, family, and diabetes communities is crucial to navigating these challenges and maintaining good health.

Conclusion

Type 1 diabetes is a complex autoimmune condition that requires careful management to prevent complications. While the cause of the disease is not fully understood, the underlying mechanism—an immune system attack on the pancreas's beta cells—is well documented. Early diagnosis, along with timely treatment and lifestyle adjustments, can help individuals with Type 1 diabetes lead healthy, fulfilling lives.

Chapter 7

Type 2 Diabetes – Insulin Resistance and Lifestyle Factors

Type 2 diabetes (T2D) is the most common form of diabetes, affecting millions of people worldwide. Unlike Type 1 diabetes, which is caused by an autoimmune attack on the insulin-producing beta cells of the pancreas, Type 2 diabetes primarily develops due to **insulin resistance** and impaired insulin secretion. Insulin resistance means that the body's cells no longer respond to insulin as effectively, leading to higher blood glucose levels. Over time, the pancreas works harder to produce more insulin to compensate, but it may not be able to keep up with the demand.

While genetics play a role in the development of Type 2 diabetes, **lifestyle factors**—such as diet, physical activity, weight management, and stress levels—have a profound impact on its onset and progression. In this chapter, we will explore how insulin resistance develops, the risk factors that contribute to Type 2 diabetes, and the lifestyle changes that can help prevent or manage the condition.

The Mechanism of Insulin Resistance

Insulin is a hormone produced by the **beta cells** of the pancreas that helps regulate blood glucose levels by allowing glucose to enter cells for energy. In individuals with Type 2 diabetes, the body becomes **insulin resistant**, meaning the cells—particularly those in muscle, fat, and the liver—become less responsive to insulin. This resistance impairs the ability of insulin to facilitate glucose uptake, leading to higher levels of glucose in the bloodstream.

As a result, the pancreas compensates by producing more insulin to try to overcome the resistance. Initially, this extra insulin may be sufficient to maintain normal blood glucose levels, but over time, the pancreas may become unable to produce enough insulin to keep blood sugar in check. This leads to **hyperglycemia** (high blood sugar), which, if left untreated, can lead to the development of Type 2 diabetes. The exact cause of insulin resistance is complex and not fully understood, but several factors—ranging from genetics to lifestyle habits—are believed to play a key role.

How Insulin Resistance Develops

The development of insulin resistance is thought to occur in stages, and the process is influenced by both **genetic predisposition** and **environmental factors**:

Genetic Predisposition: Some individuals are genetically predisposed to insulin resistance, meaning they are more likely to develop Type 2 diabetes if they have a family history of the condition. This genetic vulnerability may involve variations in genes that regulate metabolism, insulin signaling, and fat storage.

1. **Obesity**: One of the most significant risk factors for insulin resistance is **obesity**, particularly excess abdominal fat. Adipose (fat) tissue, especially visceral fat (fat around the internal organs), releases hormones and inflammatory cytokines that interfere with insulin signaling. This causes the body to become less sensitive to insulin, increasing the risk of insulin resistance. As fat stores grow, the liver and muscle cells may become less able to absorb glucose, exacerbating the problem.

2. **Physical Inactivity**: A sedentary lifestyle is another major contributor to insulin resistance. Regular physical activity helps improve insulin sensitivity, allowing the body to use glucose more efficiently. When people are inactive, their muscles become less efficient at taking up glucose from the bloodstream, leading to an increased risk of insulin resistance.

3. **Poor Diet**: Diets high in **refined carbohydrates**, **added sugars**, and **saturated fats** are linked to the development of insulin resistance. These types of foods cause rapid spikes in blood sugar levels, leading to increased demand for insulin. Over time, this constant demand for insulin can overwhelm the body, contributing to insulin resistance. Conversely, diets rich in fiber, whole grains, healthy fats, and lean proteins can help improve insulin sensitivity.

4. **Chronic Stress**: Stress, particularly long-term stress, can also contribute to insulin resistance. Stress hormones such as **cortisol** can raise blood glucose levels and make the body less responsive to insulin. Chronic stress can lead to poor eating habits, reduced physical activity, and weight gain, all of which further increase the risk of developing Type 2 diabetes.

5. **Age and Hormonal Changes**: As individuals age, their risk of developing Type 2 diabetes increases. Older adults are more likely to develop insulin resistance because of changes in body composition, such as increased fat mass and decreased muscle mass. Additionally, hormonal changes related to aging, such as a decrease in growth hormone levels, can also contribute to insulin resistance.

Key Risk Factors for Type 2 Diabetes

Several factors increase the likelihood of developing Type 2 diabetes. Some of these are **modifiable**, meaning they can be changed with lifestyle adjustments, while others are **non-modifiable**, meaning they cannot be altered. Understanding these risk factors can help individuals take preventive steps to reduce their risk.

Modifiable Risk Factors

1. **Obesity and Overweight**: Obesity is the single most important modifiable risk factor for Type 2 diabetes. Excess body fat, particularly abdominal fat, increases insulin resistance. Weight loss through diet and exercise can significantly improve insulin sensitivity and reduce the risk of developing diabetes.

2. **Physical Inactivity**: Sedentary behavior contributes to insulin resistance. People who do not engage in regular physical activity are at a much higher risk for Type 2 diabetes. Exercise helps the body use glucose more effectively and can prevent or delay the onset of diabetes.

3. **Unhealthy Diet**: A diet high in refined sugars, processed foods, and unhealthy fats increases the risk of Type 2 diabetes. Consuming a diet rich in fruits, vegetables, whole grains, lean proteins, and healthy fats can improve insulin sensitivity and reduce blood sugar levels.

4. **High Blood Pressure**: Hypertension (high blood pressure) is common in people with Type 2 diabetes. The presence of both conditions increases the risk of cardiovascular disease. Managing blood pressure through medication, diet, and lifestyle changes is essential for preventing complications.

5. **High Cholesterol**: High levels of **low-density lipoprotein (LDL)** cholesterol and triglycerides are common in people with Type 2 diabetes. Improving cholesterol levels through diet, exercise, and medication can help reduce the risk of heart disease and other complications.

6. **Sleep Apnea**: Sleep apnea, a condition in which breathing is repeatedly interrupted during sleep, has been linked to insulin resistance and Type 2 diabetes. Treating sleep apnea can improve blood sugar control.

Non-Modifiable Risk Factors

1. **Age**: The risk of Type 2 diabetes increases with age, particularly after the age of 45. As people age, they often become less active and may gain weight, both of which contribute to the development of insulin resistance.

2. **Family History**: Having a first-degree relative (parent or sibling) with Type 2 diabetes significantly increases the risk of developing the condition. While genetic predisposition cannot be changed, individuals with a family history of Type 2 diabetes can take preventive steps by maintaining a healthy lifestyle.

3. **Ethnicity**: Certain ethnic groups are at a higher risk for Type 2 diabetes. These include **African Americans, Hispanic Americans, Native Americans**, and **Asian Americans**. While genetics and lifestyle factors contribute to this higher risk, early screening and lifestyle modifications can help mitigate the impact.

4. **Gestational Diabetes**: Women who have had **gestational diabetes** during pregnancy are at a higher risk of developing Type 2 diabetes later in life. After pregnancy, these women should maintain a healthy weight, stay active, and monitor their blood sugar levels.

5. **Polycystic Ovary Syndrome (PCOS)**: Women with **PCOS** often experience insulin resistance and have a higher risk of developing Type 2 diabetes. Managing weight, engaging in physical activity, and, when necessary, using medication can help reduce this risk.

Symptoms and Diagnosis of Type 2 Diabetes

The symptoms of Type 2 diabetes develop gradually, and many individuals may not notice them at first. Common symptoms include:

- **Increased thirst** and frequent urination
- **Fatigue** or feeling unusually tired
- **Blurred vision**
- **Slow-healing sores** or frequent infections
- **Numbness or tingling** in the hands or feet
- **Unexplained weight loss** (though more common in Type 1 diabetes, some people with Type 2 may experience weight loss due to poor glucose regulation)

Because the symptoms are often subtle or overlooked, many people with Type 2 diabetes may not be diagnosed until they develop complications. To diagnose Type 2 diabetes, doctors may perform the following tests:

- **Fasting blood glucose test**: A fasting blood glucose level of **126 mg/dL (7.0 mmol/L)** or higher suggests Type 2 diabetes.
- **Oral glucose tolerance test (OGTT)**: This test measures the body's response to a glucose challenge. A blood sugar level of **200 mg/dL (11.1 mmol/L)** or higher two hours after drinking the glucose solution is diagnostic for diabetes.
- **Hemoglobin A1c test**: An HbA1c level of **6.5%** or higher indicates diabetes.

Prevention and Management of Type 2 Diabetes

The most effective way to prevent or manage Type 2 diabetes is through lifestyle changes. Here are some key strategies:

1. **Weight Management**: Losing even a small amount of weight—5-10% of body weight—can significantly improve insulin sensitivity and reduce the risk of Type 2 diabetes. Maintaining a healthy weight is essential for both preventing and managing the condition.

2. **Physical Activity**: Regular physical activity is one of the most effective ways to improve insulin sensitivity. Aim for at least **150 minutes of moderate-intensity exercise** each week, such as walking, swimming, or cycling.

3. **Healthy Eating**: A balanced diet rich in whole grains, fruits, vegetables, lean proteins, and healthy fats is crucial. Avoid processed foods and limit the intake of sugary drinks, refined carbs, and unhealthy fats.

4. **Stress Management**: Chronic stress can exacerbate insulin resistance. Practicing relaxation techniques such as deep breathing, meditation, and yoga can help manage stress levels.

5. **Medication**: For individuals who have been diagnosed with Type 2 diabetes, medications such as **metformin** may be prescribed to help improve insulin sensitivity and regulate blood sugar levels. In some cases, insulin therapy may be necessary.

6. **Regular Monitoring**: Monitoring blood sugar levels regularly is essential for managing Type 2 diabetes. Continuous glucose monitoring (CGM) devices or periodic blood tests can help track fluctuations and make adjustments to treatment as needed.

Conclusion

Type 2 diabetes is primarily a result of insulin resistance and lifestyle factors, with genetics playing a secondary role. The condition is preventable and manageable with lifestyle changes, including weight management, increased physical activity, and healthy eating habits. By understanding the mechanisms behind insulin resistance and identifying risk factors, individuals can take proactive steps to reduce their risk of developing Type 2 diabetes and improve their overall health.

Chapter 8

Gestational Diabetes – Diabetes During Pregnancy

Gestational diabetes (GDM) is a form of diabetes that develops during pregnancy and affects how a woman's body processes glucose. Unlike Type 1 and Type 2 diabetes, which are chronic conditions, gestational diabetes occurs only during pregnancy, typically in the second or third trimester. Although GDM often resolves after childbirth, it carries significant risks for both the mother and the baby if not carefully managed. In this chapter, we will explore the causes of gestational diabetes, the risks involved, how it is managed, and the long-term implications for both mother and child.

What is Gestational Diabetes?

Gestational diabetes is a condition in which a woman experiences **high blood sugar levels** during pregnancy. It typically develops when the body cannot produce enough insulin to meet the increased needs during pregnancy. Insulin is a hormone that helps regulate blood glucose levels by allowing glucose to enter cells for energy. During pregnancy, hormonal changes can lead to **insulin resistance**, meaning that the body's cells become less responsive to insulin, resulting in higher blood glucose levels.

In normal pregnancies, the pancreas increases insulin production to compensate for this insulin resistance. However, in some women, the pancreas is unable to produce enough insulin to overcome this resistance, leading to **gestational diabetes**. If left untreated, gestational diabetes can lead to complications for both the mother and the baby.

Causes of Gestational Diabetes

The exact cause of gestational diabetes is not completely understood, but several factors contribute to its development:

1. **Hormonal Changes in Pregnancy**: During pregnancy, the body undergoes significant hormonal changes, and certain hormones produced by the placenta, such as **human placental lactogen (HPL)**, **cortisol**, and **progesterone**, can increase insulin resistance. While these hormones help ensure adequate glucose supply for the growing baby, they can also reduce the efficiency of insulin in the mother's body.

2. **Insulin Resistance**: As pregnancy progresses, the placenta releases hormones that interfere with the action of insulin, making the mother's cells less responsive to it. This leads to insulin resistance, which causes higher blood glucose levels.

3. **Increased Insulin Production**: In response to insulin resistance, the pancreas must work harder to produce enough insulin to regulate blood sugar. In some women, the pancreas is unable to keep up with the increased demand, leading to the development of **gestational diabetes**.

4. **Genetic and Lifestyle Factors**: Women with a family history of diabetes, especially Type 2 diabetes, are at a higher risk of developing gestational diabetes. Additionally, **obesity**, **sedentary lifestyle**, and **poor nutrition** can increase the likelihood of developing the condition. Ethnicity also plays a role, with women of African American, Hispanic, Native American, and Asian American descent having a higher risk.

Risk Factors for Gestational Diabetes

Several factors can increase a woman's risk of developing gestational diabetes during pregnancy. These include:

- **Obesity**: Being overweight or obese before pregnancy is a significant risk factor for gestational diabetes. Fat cells produce hormones that can increase insulin resistance, making it more difficult for the body to regulate blood sugar levels.
- **Age**: Women over the age of **25** are more likely to develop gestational diabetes, though the risk increases significantly after the age of 35.
- **Family History of Diabetes**: Women with a **family history** of diabetes (Type 1 or Type 2) are more likely to develop gestational diabetes.
- **Previous Gestational Diabetes**: Women who have had gestational diabetes during a previous pregnancy are at a higher risk of developing it again in subsequent pregnancies.
- **Ethnic Background**: Certain ethnic groups, including **African American**, **Hispanic**, **Native American**, and **Asian American** women, are more likely to develop gestational diabetes.
- **Polycystic Ovary Syndrome (PCOS)**: Women with **PCOS** are more likely to develop gestational diabetes due to the insulin resistance often associated with the condition.
- **High Blood Pressure**: Having **hypertension** or high blood pressure before or during pregnancy increases the risk of gestational diabetes.
- **Large Baby in Previous Pregnancy**: Women who have given birth to a baby weighing more than **9 pounds** (4.1 kg) are at a higher risk of developing gestational diabetes in subsequent pregnancies.

Symptoms of Gestational Diabetes

Gestational diabetes often develops without noticeable symptoms, which is why regular screening during pregnancy is so important. When symptoms do occur, they may include:

- **Increased thirst** (polydipsia)

- **Frequent urination** (polyuria)
- **Fatigue**
- **Blurred vision**
- **Frequent infections**, particularly urinary tract infections (UTIs)
- **Nausea**

Because the symptoms of gestational diabetes are often mild or overlooked, it's crucial for pregnant women to undergo routine screening for gestational diabetes, typically between **24 and 28 weeks** of pregnancy.

Diagnosis of Gestational Diabetes

Gestational diabetes is diagnosed through screening tests, typically performed between **24 and 28 weeks** of pregnancy. The **oral glucose tolerance test (OGTT)** is the standard test used to diagnose the condition. During this test, the woman will drink a sugary solution, and her blood sugar levels will be measured at intervals after ingestion. The test is done in two parts:

1. **Initial screening**: Women are typically given a **50-gram glucose solution** and have their blood sugar checked one hour later. If the blood glucose level exceeds **140 mg/dL** (7.8 mmol/L), further testing is needed.

2. **Diagnostic test**: The **75-gram oral glucose tolerance test** is administered, and blood glucose levels are measured at fasting and at 1, 2, and 3-hour intervals. If two or more of the following levels are exceeded, a diagnosis of gestational diabetes is made:

   - Fasting blood glucose: **92 mg/dL (5.1 mmol/L) or higher**
   - 1-hour blood glucose: **180 mg/dL (10.0 mmol/L) or higher**
   - 2-hour blood glucose: **153 mg/dL (8.5 mmol/L) or higher**

If gestational diabetes is diagnosed, the woman will be monitored more closely throughout her pregnancy.

Management of Gestational Diabetes

Gestational diabetes is manageable with lifestyle changes and, in some cases, medication. The primary goals of managing gestational diabetes are to control blood sugar levels, reduce the risk of complications, and ensure the health of both mother and baby. The treatment approach includes:

1. **Dietary Modifications**: A **balanced diet** is key in managing gestational diabetes. A registered dietitian can help develop a meal plan that emphasizes:
   - **Complex carbohydrates** (whole grains, legumes, vegetables)
   - **Lean proteins** (chicken, fish, tofu, beans)
   - **Healthy fats** (avocado, olive oil, nuts)
   - **Fiber-rich foods** (fruits, vegetables, whole grains) A healthy diet helps stabilize blood sugar levels and provides essential nutrients for both the mother and the developing baby.

2. **Physical Activity**: Regular **exercise** helps improve insulin sensitivity and can lower blood sugar levels. For women with gestational diabetes, safe activities such as walking, swimming, and prenatal yoga are encouraged. Exercise can also help with weight management and prevent excessive weight gain during pregnancy.

3. **Blood Sugar Monitoring**: Women with gestational diabetes are often instructed to monitor their blood sugar levels regularly, typically several times a day. This helps track how food, exercise, and medication (if prescribed) affect blood glucose levels.

4. **Insulin Therapy**: In some cases, diet and exercise alone are not enough to control blood sugar levels. If blood sugar remains high, insulin injections may be prescribed to help regulate blood sugar. Unlike oral medications, insulin does not cross the placenta and is considered safe during pregnancy.

5. **Oral Medications**: Although insulin is the most common treatment, some women may be prescribed oral medications, such as **metformin** or **glyburide**, if they are unable to control blood sugar levels through diet and exercise. These medications help the body use insulin more effectively.

6. **Close Monitoring of Fetal Health**: Regular ultrasounds and fetal monitoring are essential to check for complications such as excessive fetal growth (macrosomia) or signs of fetal distress. Close monitoring helps doctors take timely action to prevent problems during labor and delivery.

Long-Term Risks for Mother and Baby

While gestational diabetes typically resolves after childbirth, it carries long-term risks for both mother and baby.

Risks for the Mother:

1. **Increased Risk of Type 2 Diabetes**: Women who have had gestational diabetes are at a significantly higher risk of developing Type 2 diabetes later in life. It is estimated that 50% of women with gestational diabetes will develop Type 2 diabetes within 5 to 10 years after pregnancy.

2. **Cardiovascular Disease**: Gestational diabetes has been linked to an increased risk of heart disease and stroke. Women who had gestational diabetes are more likely to develop high blood pressure, high cholesterol, and other risk factors for cardiovascular disease.

3. **Future Pregnancies**: Women who have had gestational diabetes are at a higher risk of developing it in future pregnancies. Therefore, they need to be closely monitored during subsequent pregnancies.

Risks for the Baby:

1. **Excessive Birth Weight (Macrosomia)**: One of the most significant risks associated with gestational diabetes is having a **large baby**. High blood sugar levels can cause the fetus to grow larger than average, increasing the likelihood of a **cesarean section** and increasing the risk of **birth injuries**.

2. **Premature Birth**: Babies born to mothers with gestational diabetes may be at a higher risk of being born prematurely. Premature birth can lead to complications such as respiratory problems and low blood sugar after birth.

3. **Low Blood Sugar (Hypoglycemia)**: After birth, babies born to mothers with gestational diabetes may experience low blood sugar (hypoglycemia). This is because their insulin production is high due to exposure to high maternal glucose levels in utero.

4. **Increased Risk of Obesity and Diabetes**: Children born to mothers with gestational diabetes are at a higher risk of becoming obese and developing Type 2 diabetes later in life.

Conclusion

Gestational diabetes is a serious condition that can lead to complications for both the mother and baby if not properly managed. While the condition usually resolves after childbirth, women with gestational diabetes are at higher risk of developing Type 2 diabetes in the future. Early detection, careful management through diet, exercise, and blood sugar monitoring, and regular prenatal care are crucial to ensuring the health of both mother and child. By taking proactive steps, women can reduce the risks of gestational diabetes and enjoy healthier pregnancies.

Chapter 9

LADA – Latent Autoimmune Diabetes in Adults

Latent Autoimmune Diabetes in Adults (LADA) is a form of diabetes that shares characteristics with both Type 1 and Type 2 diabetes but is often misdiagnosed as Type 2 due to its slower progression and adult onset. LADA is considered a **hybrid** form of diabetes, combining autoimmune destruction of insulin-producing beta cells in the pancreas (similar to Type 1 diabetes) with features of insulin resistance (more common in Type 2 diabetes). This chapter will explore the nature of LADA, how it differs from Type 1 and Type 2 diabetes, and the challenges in diagnosing and managing this lesser-known form of diabetes.

What is LADA?

LADA, also known as **Type 1.5 diabetes**, is a relatively recently recognized form of diabetes that typically develops in **adults** over the age of 30. Like Type 1 diabetes, LADA is an **autoimmune condition** in which the body's immune system attacks and destroys the insulin-producing beta cells in the pancreas. However, unlike Type 1 diabetes, which typically presents in childhood or adolescence, LADA usually develops more gradually and manifests later in life.

The progression of LADA is typically slower than that of Type 1 diabetes, which means that people with LADA may still produce some insulin at first and may not require insulin therapy immediately. In fact, for the first few years, the disease can resemble **Type 2 diabetes**, with initial management involving oral medications like **metformin** to control blood sugar levels. However, as the autoimmune process continues, the body's ability to produce insulin declines, leading to the eventual need for **insulin injections**—a hallmark of Type 1 diabetes.

Because LADA is often initially misdiagnosed as Type 2 diabetes, it can go untreated for several years, which can lead to serious complications such as cardiovascular disease, kidney damage, and neuropathy.

How LADA Differs from Type 1 and Type 2 Diabetes

While LADA shares some characteristics with both Type 1 and Type 2 diabetes, it is distinct from both conditions in several ways:

1. **Autoimmune Component**: Like **Type 1 diabetes**, LADA is an autoimmune disorder. In Type 1 diabetes, the body's immune system attacks and destroys the beta cells in the pancreas that produce insulin, leading to absolute insulin deficiency. In LADA, a similar autoimmune process occurs, but it typically happens at a much slower pace, allowing for some beta cell function to remain for a period of time. However, the eventual progression of LADA typically leads to complete insulin dependency.

2. **Age of Onset**: LADA typically affects **adults** aged 30 and older, which is different from Type 1 diabetes, which usually develops in childhood or adolescence. Type 2 diabetes, on the other hand, is most common in individuals over the age of 40, though it is increasingly being diagnosed in younger populations due to the rise in obesity and sedentary lifestyles.

3. **Insulin Resistance**: One of the defining features of **Type 2 diabetes** is insulin resistance, where the body's cells become less responsive to insulin, requiring the pancreas to produce more insulin to maintain normal blood glucose levels. People with Type 2 diabetes may initially manage their condition with oral medications and lifestyle changes.

While LADA does involve some insulin resistance, it is not the primary feature of the condition. People with LADA typically experience a gradual decline in insulin production due to the autoimmune destruction of beta cells, making insulin therapy inevitable as the disease progresses.

4. **Beta Cell Function**: In **Type 1 diabetes**, beta cell function is rapidly destroyed after the autoimmune attack, leading to immediate insulin dependence. In contrast, people with LADA may have partial beta cell function for years before insulin therapy becomes necessary. This means that initial treatment may involve oral medications, and the progression to insulin dependency can take several years.

5. **Initial Treatment**: **Type 2 diabetes** is often managed with lifestyle changes, oral medications, and sometimes insulin therapy. LADA, however, is initially treated with oral medications, similar to Type 2 diabetes. Over time, however, as beta cell function declines, patients with LADA eventually require **insulin injections** to maintain blood sugar control, much like individuals with Type 1 diabetes.

Challenges in Diagnosing LADA

Diagnosing LADA can be particularly challenging due to its gradual onset and the overlap of symptoms with Type 2 diabetes. The initial presentation of LADA may be similar to Type 2 diabetes, with symptoms such as:

- Increased thirst
- Frequent urination
- Fatigue
- Blurred vision

However, because LADA develops more slowly than Type 1 diabetes and often occurs in adults who are overweight or have a family history of

Type 2 diabetes, doctors may initially misdiagnose the condition as Type 2 diabetes. This can delay appropriate treatment, which may lead to poor blood glucose control and long-term complications.

Some of the key diagnostic challenges include:

1. **Age of Onset**: Since LADA usually affects adults aged 30 and older, it can be mistaken for Type 2 diabetes, which is most common in older individuals. The age of onset is one of the most significant factors in diagnosing LADA, as **Type 1 diabetes** typically develops in childhood or adolescence.

2. **Gradual Progression**: Unlike Type 1 diabetes, which presents rapidly with severe symptoms, LADA progresses slowly over several years. This means that blood glucose levels may be elevated, but not to the point where insulin therapy is immediately necessary. Therefore, it may not trigger the usual alarms that would lead to a diagnosis of Type 1 diabetes.

3. **Misinterpretation of Symptoms**: Many of the early symptoms of LADA—such as increased thirst, fatigue, and blurred vision—are common to both **Type 2 diabetes** and **LADA**. Therefore, doctors may initially prescribe oral medications such as metformin, which may temporarily control blood sugar levels, but fail to address the underlying autoimmune destruction of the beta cells.

4. **Autoimmune Testing**: To properly diagnose LADA, a doctor may need to perform **autoantibody tests**, which detect the presence of antibodies that attack beta cells in the pancreas. These tests include the **GAD (Glutamic acid decarboxylase)** antibody test, which is commonly elevated in individuals with LADA. The presence of GAD antibodies in combination with elevated blood glucose levels and gradual insulin dependence suggests that LADA is the underlying cause. However, not

all people with LADA test positive for these autoantibodies, further complicating the diagnosis.

5. **Differentiating from Type 2 Diabetes**: In many cases, LADA is misdiagnosed as Type 2 diabetes, and treatment with oral medications such as metformin may initially control blood sugar levels. However, as beta cell function declines, patients with LADA may require insulin therapy much sooner than expected. Misdiagnosing LADA as Type 2 diabetes can lead to delayed initiation of insulin therapy, which can increase the risk of complications.

Management of LADA

Managing LADA can be difficult due to its progressive nature and the need for both autoimmune and metabolic control. Early in the disease, treatment may involve lifestyle changes and oral medications, while later stages will require insulin therapy.

1. **Lifestyle Modifications**: Like other forms of diabetes, **dietary changes** and **physical activity** play a critical role in managing LADA. A healthy, balanced diet with a focus on **low glycemic index foods** and **whole grains** can help regulate blood sugar levels. Regular exercise, especially strength training and aerobic exercise, can improve insulin sensitivity and help maintain a healthy weight, which is important for managing insulin resistance in the early stages of LADA.

2. **Oral Medications**: In the early stages of LADA, doctors may prescribe oral medications such as **metformin, sulfonylureas,** or **DPP-4 inhibitors** to help control blood sugar levels. These medications work by improving insulin sensitivity, stimulating the pancreas to produce more insulin, or preventing the breakdown of incretin hormones that help

regulate blood sugar. However, as the disease progresses and beta cell function deteriorates, these medications become less effective, and insulin therapy will eventually be necessary.

3. **Insulin Therapy**: As beta cell function declines, insulin injections become essential for managing LADA. Insulin therapy in LADA is similar to Type 1 diabetes, where individuals may need to use **rapid-acting insulin** before meals and **long-acting insulin** to control blood sugar between meals and overnight. Some individuals may benefit from an **insulin pump** or **continuous glucose monitoring (CGM)** to help keep their blood sugar levels within target ranges.

4. **Monitoring and Medical Support**: Because LADA progresses over several years, regular monitoring of **blood glucose levels** is crucial. People with LADA should have regular visits with their healthcare providers to assess insulin needs and to monitor for complications such as diabetic retinopathy, neuropathy, and kidney disease. **Autoantibody tests** may be performed periodically to assess the degree of autoimmune involvement.

5. **Education and Support**: Due to the complexity of managing LADA, people diagnosed with the condition often benefit from **diabetes education** and **support groups**. Learning about the disease, understanding how to manage blood sugar levels, and coping with the emotional and psychological aspects of living with a chronic condition are critical components of care.

Long-Term Outlook for People with LADA

The long-term outlook for people with LADA is generally positive if the condition is properly managed. However, because LADA involves autoimmune destruction of the beta cells, individuals with this form of diabetes will eventually require insulin therapy. Early diagnosis and appropriate management can help prevent complications and improve quality of life.

People with LADA also need to be vigilant about their long-term health, as they are at a higher risk of developing complications such as **cardiovascular disease**, **kidney damage**, and **neuropathy**. Maintaining good blood sugar control, adhering to a healthy lifestyle, and working closely with healthcare providers are key to living a healthy life with LADA.

Conclusion

LADA, or Latent Autoimmune Diabetes in Adults, is a complex and often misdiagnosed form of diabetes that combines elements of both Type 1 and Type 2 diabetes. The gradual onset and autoimmune nature of the condition present unique challenges in diagnosis and management. However, with appropriate recognition and treatment, individuals with LADA can live healthy, fulfilling lives.

Early intervention with lifestyle changes, medications, and insulin therapy is essential to managing the disease and preventing complications. As awareness of LADA continues to grow, more people will be able to receive the correct diagnosis and care, improving outcomes and quality of life.

Chapter 10

MODY – Maturity-Onset Diabetes of the Young

Maturity-Onset Diabetes of the Young (MODY) is a rare form of diabetes that is caused by genetic mutations and typically presents in adolescents or young adults. Unlike the more common types of diabetes—Type 1 and Type 2—MODY is not primarily influenced by lifestyle factors such as obesity or physical inactivity, and it is not an autoimmune condition. Instead, MODY is an inherited disorder that is due to specific genetic mutations that affect the body's ability to regulate blood glucose. In this chapter, we will explore the genetic causes and characteristics of MODY, how it differs from Type 1 and Type 2 diabetes, and the importance of genetic testing in diagnosing and managing the condition.

What is MODY?

MODY is a form of **genetically determined diabetes** that typically manifests in **children, adolescents**, or young adults, usually before the age of **25**. It is caused by mutations in a single gene that affects the body's ability to produce or utilize insulin effectively. Unlike Type 1 and Type 2 diabetes, which are influenced by multiple genetic and environmental factors, MODY is typically the result of a **monogenic** defect—that is, a mutation in a **single gene** that directly affects insulin production, secretion, or action.

MODY is considered an **inherited** form of diabetes, meaning it runs in families and is passed down through generations in an **autosomal dominant** pattern. This means that if one parent carries the defective gene, there is a 50% chance that each child will inherit it and potentially develop MODY.

Over the years, scientists have identified multiple types of MODY, each caused by mutations in different genes. The specific gene mutation determines the characteristics and management of the condition, but the hallmark of MODY is that it presents **early in life**, often with mild to moderate hyperglycemia (high blood sugar levels), and can often be managed with oral medications rather than insulin injections.

Genetic Causes of MODY

The genetic cause of MODY lies in mutations in any one of several genes involved in insulin production or secretion. These mutations typically result in impaired insulin release from the pancreas, leading to higher blood glucose levels. Although there are many forms of MODY, the most common types are:

1. **MODY 1 (HNF4A)**:
   - This form of MODY is caused by a mutation in the **HNF4A** gene (hepatocyte nuclear factor 4-alpha), which plays a role in regulating insulin production in the pancreas. Individuals with MODY 1 typically experience **early-onset diabetes**, often before the age of 25. This form of MODY usually responds well to oral medications like **sulfonylureas**, which stimulate insulin release from the pancreas.

2. **MODY 2 (GCK)**:
   - Caused by a mutation in the **GCK** gene (glucokinase), which regulates glucose sensing in the pancreas, liver, and other tissues. People with MODY 2 often have mild, stable hyperglycemia that is

usually not associated with the development of complications. This form of MODY tends to be less severe than other forms and may not require treatment beyond occasional monitoring of blood sugar levels.

3. **MODY 3 (HNF1A)**:
   - This is the most common form of MODY, caused by mutations in the **HNF1A** gene (hepatocyte nuclear factor 1-alpha). Like MODY 1, MODY 3 leads to **impaired insulin secretion**, but it can also affect other organs, such as the kidneys and liver. People with MODY 3 may have early-onset diabetes that can often be managed with **oral medications**, such as sulfonylureas, though some individuals may require insulin as the condition progresses.

4. **MODY 4 (IPF1)**:
   - This rare form of MODY is caused by mutations in the **IPF1** gene (insulin promoter factor 1), which is critical for normal insulin gene expression and beta cell function. MODY 4 can cause a more severe form of diabetes and often requires insulin therapy.

5. **MODY 5 (HNF1B)**:
   - MODY 5 results from mutations in the **HNF1B** gene and is associated with both **diabetes and other kidney abnormalities**, such as renal cysts and structural kidney problems. The diabetes in MODY 5 may be more difficult to manage, often requiring insulin therapy, and kidney function may also be compromised over time.

6. **MODY 6, 7, and 8**:
   - These are rare forms of MODY caused by mutations in various other genes, including **NEUROD1** and **KLF11**. Each of these forms of MODY is distinct and often requires specialized

treatment, though they share similar characteristics in terms of early-onset diabetes and impaired insulin secretion.

The genetic mutations in these various forms of MODY result in problems with the insulin secretion process, either causing too little insulin to be produced or making the body's insulin less effective in controlling blood sugar. The onset of the condition usually occurs in adolescence or early adulthood, and affected individuals may not require insulin treatment in the early stages of the disease.

How MODY Differs from Type 1 and Type 2 Diabetes

While MODY shares certain characteristics with both **Type 1** and **Type 2** diabetes, it is a distinct form of the disease. Understanding the differences between MODY, Type 1, and Type 2 diabetes is crucial for proper diagnosis and treatment.

1. **Age of Onset**:
   - **Type 1 diabetes** typically develops in **childhood** or **adolescence** and is characterized by rapid onset and severe insulin deficiency.
   - **Type 2 diabetes** usually develops in **adults**, often after the age of **40**, and is primarily associated with **insulin resistance** rather than an autoimmune attack on beta cells.
   - **MODY**, on the other hand, typically presents **before the age of 25** and can affect children, teenagers, and young adults. It is important to note that MODY can often be misdiagnosed as Type 1 or Type 2 diabetes because it presents in a similar age group and has overlapping symptoms.

2. **Genetic Basis**:

- **Type 1 diabetes** is an **autoimmune** condition where the immune system attacks and destroys the insulin-producing beta cells in the pancreas. It is often diagnosed suddenly with severe symptoms and requires insulin therapy from the outset.
- **Type 2 diabetes** is primarily driven by **insulin resistance**, where the body's cells become less responsive to insulin. It is strongly influenced by lifestyle factors, such as **obesity** and **physical inactivity**, and is often treated initially with **oral medications** or lifestyle changes.
- **MODY**, in contrast, is caused by **genetic mutations** in a single gene. It is inherited in an **autosomal dominant** pattern, meaning that one affected parent can pass the mutation down to their children. The presence of MODY in multiple family members is a key clue to its diagnosis.

3. **Insulin Dependence**:
   - **Type 1 diabetes** leads to **absolute insulin deficiency**, meaning that individuals with Type 1 diabetes must rely on insulin therapy for the rest of their lives.
   - **Type 2 diabetes** is often initially managed with **oral medications** and lifestyle changes. Insulin is typically not required until the later stages of the disease when beta cell function declines.
   - **MODY** typically begins with **mild to moderate hyperglycemia** that may be controlled with **oral medications** like sulfonylureas. As the disease progresses, some individuals with MODY may eventually require **insulin therapy**, although this occurs much later than in Type 1 diabetes.

4. **Management**:

- o **Type 1 diabetes** requires lifelong **insulin therapy**, as the pancreas can no longer produce insulin.
- o **Type 2 diabetes** is often managed with **oral medications**, lifestyle changes, and in some cases, insulin therapy.
- o **MODY**, depending on the genetic mutation, may respond to **oral medications**, particularly **sulfonylureas**, which stimulate the pancreas to release more insulin. In some cases, insulin therapy may be necessary as the condition progresses.

The Importance of Genetic Testing

Because MODY is caused by specific genetic mutations, **genetic testing** plays a critical role in its diagnosis. Genetic testing can confirm whether an individual has a mutation in one of the genes associated with MODY, allowing for a more accurate diagnosis and helping to differentiate MODY from other forms of diabetes.

Some of the key reasons why genetic testing is important in MODY include:

1. **Accurate Diagnosis**: Genetic testing can identify mutations in specific genes (such as **HNF4A, GCK**, or **HNF1A**) that are responsible for MODY. This can help clarify whether a person has MODY or another form of diabetes, such as Type 1 or Type 2, which may have similar symptoms but requires different treatment strategies.

2. **Guiding Treatment**: Identifying the specific type of MODY can help healthcare providers determine the most appropriate treatment plan. For example, people with MODY 1 or MODY 3 may respond well to **sulfonylureas**, while others with different types of MODY may require

insulin therapy. Genetic testing helps avoid unnecessary insulin treatment in cases where oral medications would be more appropriate.

3. **Family Screening**: Since MODY is inherited in an autosomal dominant pattern, genetic testing can help identify other family members who may be at risk for developing the condition. This allows for early diagnosis and intervention, reducing the risk of complications.

4. **Preventing Misdiagnosis**: Without genetic testing, MODY can often be misdiagnosed as Type 1 or Type 2 diabetes. This can lead to inappropriate treatments and delays in managing the disease. For example, people with MODY may be incorrectly prescribed insulin therapy if their condition is initially mistaken for Type 1 diabetes.

Conclusion

Maturity-Onset Diabetes of the Young (MODY) is a genetically determined form of diabetes that presents in adolescents or young adults and is caused by mutations in a single gene that affects insulin production and secretion. While MODY shares some characteristics with Type 1 and Type 2 diabetes, it is a distinct form of diabetes that requires specific genetic testing for diagnosis and management.

Early identification of MODY is crucial for providing the right treatment and preventing complications. Genetic testing not only ensures accurate diagnosis but also helps guide treatment decisions and enables family members to be screened for the condition. Understanding the genetic basis of MODY can lead to better care and outcomes for individuals living with this unique form of diabetes.

Chapter 11

Other Rare Forms of Diabetes

Diabetes is commonly categorized into three main types: Type 1, Type 2, and gestational diabetes. However, there are also several rare forms of diabetes that are less well-known but can have significant implications for those affected. These rare types often present unique challenges in terms of diagnosis, treatment, and management. In this chapter, we will explore some of the lesser-known forms of diabetes, including **Wolfram Syndrome**, **Neonatal Diabetes**, and **Cystic Fibrosis-related Diabetes**, among others. Understanding these rarer conditions is crucial for early diagnosis and proper management, as they often require specialized care.

Wolfram Syndrome: A Complex Genetic Disorder

Wolfram Syndrome, also known as DIDMOAD syndrome (Diabetes Insipidus, Diabetes Mellitus, Optic Atrophy, and Deafness), is a rare **genetic disorder** that typically manifests in childhood or adolescence. It is caused by mutations in the **WFS1** gene, which is responsible for producing a protein involved in the function of the **endoplasmic reticulum** in cells. This condition is inherited in an **autosomal recessive** manner, meaning that an individual must inherit two copies of the mutated gene—one from each parent—in order to develop Wolfram Syndrome.

Wolfram syndrome presents with a combination of symptoms that can vary in severity, but the hallmark features include:

- **Type 1 Diabetes**: Affected individuals typically develop **insulin-dependent diabetes** at a young age, usually before the age of 15. The autoimmune destruction of insulin-producing beta cells in the pancreas leads to the need for lifelong insulin therapy.

- **Optic Atrophy**: This is another prominent feature of Wolfram syndrome, leading to **progressive vision loss** due to the degeneration of the optic nerve. It often begins in childhood and can lead to complete blindness in adulthood.

- **Deafness**: Sensorineural hearing loss is common in Wolfram syndrome, typically presenting in childhood and worsening over time.

- **Diabetes Insipidus**: This is a condition that causes excessive thirst and urination due to problems with the kidneys' ability to concentrate urine. It is often one of the earliest signs of Wolfram syndrome.

- **Neurological Issues**: Other neurological symptoms may include **ataxia** (lack of coordination), **dysphagia** (difficulty swallowing), and **cognitive impairment**.

While Wolfram syndrome is rare, it is essential to recognize the syndrome early in order to manage the symptoms and improve quality of life. Diabetes management for individuals with Wolfram syndrome is similar to that for Type 1 diabetes, with insulin therapy being a cornerstone of treatment. Other symptoms, such as hearing loss and vision impairment, require supportive interventions, and management often involves a multidisciplinary team of specialists, including endocrinologists, audiologists, ophthalmologists, and neurologists.

Neonatal Diabetes: Diabetes in Infancy

Neonatal Diabetes Mellitus (NDM) is a rare form of diabetes that occurs in **infants younger than 6 months** old. Unlike the more common forms of diabetes, which develop in older children or adults, neonatal diabetes is not autoimmune in nature and is often caused by **genetic mutations** affecting insulin production or secretion. Neonatal diabetes is distinct from Type 1 diabetes in that it is not due to an autoimmune attack on the pancreas, but rather to **defects in the insulin gene** or other genes involved in the regulation of insulin production.

The condition is **genetically determined**, and the mutations most commonly affect genes like **KCNJ11**, which codes for a potassium channel in the pancreas that plays a crucial role in insulin release. There are two main forms of neonatal diabetes:

- **Transitory Neonatal Diabetes**: In some cases, neonatal diabetes may resolve on its own in infancy, only to recur in adolescence or adulthood. This form is often associated with **chromosomal abnormalities** and can be managed with insulin during the period of active disease.

- **Permanent Neonatal Diabetes**: In other cases, neonatal diabetes is a **lifelong condition** that requires **insulin therapy** for the rest of the individual's life. This form is caused by mutations in genes responsible for insulin secretion or processing, and it may be managed with oral medications in some cases. However, **insulin therapy** remains the primary treatment.

Diagnosis of neonatal diabetes involves detecting **elevated blood glucose levels** in infants who present with symptoms such as **poor feeding, failure to thrive**, and **excessive urination**. Genetic testing can help pinpoint the underlying cause of the disease, allowing for personalized treatment plans. In some cases, genetic testing can reveal **KCNJ11 mutations** or **ABCC8 mutations**, both of which are associated with neonatal diabetes.

Management of neonatal diabetes requires careful monitoring of blood sugar levels and, in most cases, insulin therapy. The prognosis is generally good if the condition is diagnosed early and appropriately managed, though long-term monitoring is essential to detect potential complications like **growth retardation** or **diabetic complications** that can arise over time.

Cystic Fibrosis-Related Diabetes (CFRD)

Cystic Fibrosis-Related Diabetes (CFRD) is the most common form of diabetes in individuals with **cystic fibrosis (CF)**, a **genetic disorder** that causes severe damage to the lungs, pancreas, and other organs. People with cystic fibrosis experience thick mucus buildup in various organs, leading to **chronic respiratory infections**, digestive issues, and damage to the insulin-producing cells of the pancreas.

CFRD shares characteristics with both **Type 1** and **Type 2 diabetes** but is considered a unique form of diabetes due to its association with cystic fibrosis. It typically develops in **adolescents or adults** with cystic fibrosis, often after the age of **10**, and it is characterized by **insulin resistance** combined with **insulin deficiency**.

- **Insulin Resistance**: Like Type 2 diabetes, CFRD involves **insulin resistance**, where the body's cells become less responsive to insulin. This is partly due to the inflammation and damage to pancreatic tissue caused by cystic fibrosis, which impairs insulin secretion.

- **Beta Cell Dysfunction**: Over time, the pancreatic cells that produce insulin may become damaged, leading to **insulin deficiency**, similar to what occurs in Type 1 diabetes.

CFRD is diagnosed through **blood glucose testing**, and **oral glucose tolerance tests** are often used to detect early stages of the disease, especially since the symptoms of CFRD can be subtle. Early signs include increased **thirst, fatigue**, and **frequent urination**, but these symptoms may be mistaken for other issues related to cystic fibrosis. Management of CFRD involves **insulin therapy**, similar to Type 1 diabetes, as individuals with CFRD often have difficulty producing enough insulin on their own. However, because insulin resistance is also a factor, healthcare providers may focus on **improving insulin sensitivity** through lifestyle changes, physical activity, and careful monitoring of blood sugar levels.

Continuous glucose monitoring (CGM) devices may be particularly useful for tracking glucose fluctuations in people with CFRD.

Other Rare Forms of Diabetes

While Wolfram syndrome, neonatal diabetes, and cystic fibrosis-related diabetes are some of the more widely recognized rare forms of diabetes, several other conditions can lead to diabetes-like symptoms, including:

- **Alström Syndrome**: This rare genetic disorder leads to progressive vision and hearing loss, **obesity**, and **diabetes**, often in childhood or adolescence. It is caused by mutations in the **ALMS1 gene**, which affects various systems in the body, including insulin secretion and glucose metabolism.

- **MODY (Maturity-Onset Diabetes of the Young)**: Discussed in Chapter 10, MODY is a **monogenic** form of diabetes caused by genetic mutations that impair insulin secretion. It typically appears in young individuals (usually before the age of 25) and is distinct from Type 1 and Type 2 diabetes. Genetic testing can help identify the specific mutation and guide treatment.

- **Prader-Willi Syndrome**: A rare genetic disorder that causes obesity, intellectual disability, and a **constant feeling of hunger** (hyperphagia). People with Prader-Willi syndrome are at increased risk for developing **Type 2 diabetes** due to their propensity to gain weight and develop insulin resistance.

- **Klinefelter Syndrome**: This genetic condition affects males and is characterized by an extra **X chromosome** (XXY). Men with Klinefelter syndrome have a higher risk of developing **Type 2 diabetes** due to insulin resistance and obesity, although they may also experience mild insulin deficiency.

- **Mitochondrial Diabetes**: Caused by mutations in the mitochondrial DNA, this form of diabetes is often passed from mother to child. It is associated with **insulin resistance** and can occur in combination with **deafness** and other mitochondrial diseases.

Conclusion

While **Type 1** and **Type 2 diabetes** are the most common forms of diabetes, numerous rare types exist that can present unique diagnostic and treatment challenges. **Wolfram syndrome, neonatal diabetes**, and **cystic fibrosis-related diabetes** are just a few examples of rare diabetes conditions that are caused by genetic mutations and require specialized care. Early diagnosis, genetic testing, and personalized treatment plans are essential for managing these rare forms of diabetes and improving the quality of life for affected individuals. As awareness of these rarer conditions grows, healthcare providers will be better equipped to recognize, diagnose, and treat these unique forms of diabetes, ensuring that individuals with these rare conditions receive the best possible care.

Chapter 12

Symptoms and Early Warning Signs

Recognizing the early symptoms and warning signs of diabetes is crucial for early diagnosis, intervention, and effective management. Diabetes, if left undiagnosed or untreated, can lead to serious complications affecting the heart, kidneys, nerves, eyes, and other vital organs. Given that diabetes manifests differently in each type, understanding the symptoms at various stages can help individuals and healthcare providers catch the disease early, before complications arise. In this chapter, we will discuss how to recognize the signs and symptoms of diabetes at different stages of the disease and explore how early presentation can vary between the different types of diabetes.

Recognizing Common Symptoms of Diabetes

The general symptoms of diabetes are caused by prolonged high blood sugar levels (hyperglycemia) and result from the body's inability to properly utilize or produce insulin. Although specific symptoms may vary between the types of diabetes, many of the early warning signs are shared across all forms. Here are some of the most common symptoms to look out for:

- **Frequent urination (polyuria)**: One of the earliest signs of uncontrolled blood sugar is excessive urination. When blood sugar levels are high, the kidneys try to remove the excess sugar by filtering it out through the urine. This leads to an increase in urine output, often requiring more frequent trips to the bathroom.

- **Increased thirst (polydipsia)**: As the body loses more fluids through frequent urination, it becomes dehydrated, leading to an increase in thirst. People with undiagnosed or poorly controlled diabetes often find themselves drinking more than usual in an attempt to quench their thirst.

- **Fatigue**: When the body is unable to properly utilize glucose due to insulin resistance or insufficient insulin production, energy levels can drop. Fatigue or constant tiredness is one of the most common early symptoms of diabetes, particularly in Type 2 diabetes, where the body becomes resistant to insulin and struggles to use glucose for energy.

- **Blurry vision**: High blood sugar levels can cause fluid to shift in and out of the lens of the eye, leading to blurred vision. This symptom often comes on gradually, but it can worsen if blood sugar remains poorly controlled over time. While blurry vision is not specific to diabetes, it is a common sign in both newly diagnosed and long-standing diabetes.

- **Unexplained weight loss**: Weight loss is more common in **Type 1 diabetes** and can occur despite an increased appetite. This happens because the body is unable to properly use glucose for energy, leading to the breakdown of fat and muscle for fuel. In **Type 2 diabetes**, weight loss is not typically an early symptom but can occur as the disease progresses, especially in people who are already overweight or obese.

- **Slow-healing sores or frequent infections**: High blood sugar can impair the immune system's ability to fight infections, leading to slow-healing wounds or recurrent infections. This can include frequent skin, urinary tract, or yeast infections.

- **Numbness or tingling in the hands and feet**: Over time, untreated or poorly controlled diabetes can damage the nerves, leading to a condition called **diabetic neuropathy**. This often presents as numbness, tingling, or a "pins and needles" sensation in the hands and feet.

While these symptoms can be indicators of diabetes, they can also be signs of other medical conditions. If you experience any of these symptoms, it's important to see a healthcare provider for evaluation and testing.

Differences in Early Presentation Across the Types of Diabetes

Although the symptoms of diabetes may overlap, the way the disease presents can differ significantly between the different types. Here's how **Type 1**, **Type 2**, **gestational diabetes**, and other forms of diabetes may present in the early stages:

Type 1 Diabetes – Rapid Onset and Severe Symptoms

Type 1 diabetes is an **autoimmune** condition where the body's immune system mistakenly attacks and destroys the insulin-producing **beta cells** in the pancreas. This leads to **absolute insulin deficiency**, meaning the body cannot produce insulin at all.

- **Rapid onset**: The symptoms of Type 1 diabetes typically develop **quickly**, over a matter of **weeks** rather than months. Often, the first signs are dramatic, and the onset of symptoms may seem sudden. In children and adolescents, this may be particularly alarming.

- **Classic symptoms**: Along with frequent urination, increased thirst, and unexplained weight loss, individuals with Type 1 diabetes may experience **nausea, vomiting**, and **abdominal pain**. This is due to the body's inability to use glucose for energy, leading to the breakdown of fat for fuel and the production of **ketones**, which can make the blood more acidic and result in a condition known as **diabetic ketoacidosis (DKA)**.

- **Diabetic Ketoacidosis (DKA)**: DKA is a life-threatening emergency that typically presents with symptoms such as deep, rapid breathing (Kussmaul respiration), fruity-smelling breath (due to the presence of acetone), confusion, and, in severe cases, unconsciousness. DKA is more common in Type 1 diabetes and may be the first sign that an individual has the condition.

Type 2 Diabetes – Slow Onset and Subtle Symptoms

Type 2 diabetes is often referred to as **insulin resistance diabetes**, as the body becomes resistant to insulin over time, and the pancreas cannot keep up with the increased demand for insulin. Initially, blood sugar levels may remain elevated, but the body tries to compensate by producing more insulin. Over time, however, the pancreas may lose its ability to produce enough insulin.

- **Gradual onset**: Unlike Type 1 diabetes, Type 2 typically develops over a much longer period, often **years**, and symptoms may be subtle or even go unnoticed. This slow progression is why many people with Type 2 diabetes are diagnosed only after they have already experienced complications.

- **Mild symptoms**: Early signs of Type 2 diabetes may include increased thirst and urination, fatigue, and frequent infections. However, many people may not experience the classic symptoms of Type 1 diabetes, such as weight loss. Some people may even feel relatively well despite having elevated blood sugar.

- **Risk factors**: Type 2 diabetes is often linked to **lifestyle factors** such as **poor diet, physical inactivity**, and **obesity**. It is also more common in people over the age of **40**, and those with a family history of diabetes are at higher risk. Because of its slow onset and subtle symptoms, people with Type 2 diabetes may not seek medical attention until they begin experiencing complications like **nerve damage, vision problems**, or **heart disease**.

Gestational Diabetes – Occurs During Pregnancy

Gestational diabetes occurs during pregnancy when the body is unable to produce enough insulin to meet the demands of both the mother and the growing fetus. While it typically resolves after delivery, gestational diabetes can increase the risk of developing Type 2 diabetes later in life.

- **Signs during pregnancy**: Gestational diabetes often has no noticeable symptoms, which is why **routine screening** is recommended for pregnant women, typically between the **24th and 28th week** of pregnancy. However, women may experience some of the general symptoms of diabetes, such as increased thirst and urination, although these symptoms are often attributed to the natural changes during pregnancy.

- **Risk factors**: Women who are **overweight**, have a family history of diabetes, are **older than 25**, or have had gestational diabetes in a previous pregnancy are at higher risk. In some cases, gestational diabetes can be detected through a **glucose tolerance test** during prenatal visits.

- **Complications**: If left untreated, gestational diabetes can lead to complications such as **pre-eclampsia, high birth weight** (which can lead to delivery complications), and an increased risk of developing Type 2 diabetes later in life for both the mother and child.

Other Forms of Diabetes – Unique Presentations

There are several rarer forms of diabetes, such as **Maturity-Onset Diabetes of the Young (MODY)**, **Latent Autoimmune Diabetes in Adults (LADA)**, and **Neonatal Diabetes**, which can present with unique early symptoms.

- **MODY**: Typically diagnosed in young adults or teenagers, MODY often presents similarly to Type 1 diabetes but may have a more gradual onset. Unlike Type 1, which is autoimmune, MODY is caused by a genetic mutation and can often be managed with oral medications.

- **LADA**: Often called "Type 1.5 diabetes," LADA is a form of autoimmune diabetes that has a slower onset than Type 1 diabetes and may be misdiagnosed as Type 2. People with LADA often present with symptoms of **insulin deficiency** in their **30s or 40s** and may not require insulin until later stages.

- **Neonatal Diabetes**: Neonatal diabetes occurs in infants under 6 months and presents with symptoms of **failure to thrive, excessive thirst**, and **urination**. It is caused by a genetic mutation rather than autoimmune destruction of beta cells, and treatment may include insulin therapy or oral medications, depending on the cause.

Conclusion

Early recognition of diabetes symptoms is crucial to prevent the progression of the disease and its associated complications. While some of the symptoms—such as frequent urination, increased thirst, and fatigue—are common across all forms of diabetes, the way the disease presents can differ depending on the type. Type 1 diabetes typically has a rapid onset with more severe symptoms, while Type 2 diabetes tends to develop gradually and may go unnoticed for years. Gestational diabetes is unique to pregnancy and often presents without noticeable symptoms, which is why regular screening is essential. Understanding these early warning signs.

Chapter 13

How Diabetes is Diagnosed

The diagnosis of diabetes is a critical first step in managing the disease and preventing complications. Early detection through routine screening, especially for those at risk, can significantly improve long-term outcomes. While there are many tools available for diagnosing diabetes, the most commonly used methods involve blood tests. These tests measure various aspects of glucose metabolism and help identify whether blood sugar levels are abnormally high, indicating the presence of diabetes.

Additionally, the growing field of **genetic testing** has brought new insights into diagnosing rare forms of diabetes, which may require specialized testing and treatment plans. This chapter will focus on the key diagnostic tests used to identify diabetes and explore how genetic testing can be a valuable tool for diagnosing less common forms of the disease.

Blood Tests for Diagnosing Diabetes

There are several primary blood tests that healthcare professionals use to diagnose diabetes. Each of these tests provides important insights into how the body processes glucose and can help identify whether an individual has diabetes or is at risk for developing the disease.

Fasting Blood Glucose Test

The **fasting blood glucose** test is one of the most commonly used diagnostic tools for detecting diabetes. It measures the level of glucose in the blood after an individual has fasted for at least **8 hours**—usually overnight. The test is simple, widely available, and effective for diagnosing both Type 1 and Type 2 diabetes.

- **Normal Range**: A fasting blood glucose level below **100 mg/dL** (5.6 mmol/L) is considered normal.
- **Pre-diabetes**: A fasting blood glucose level between **100 mg/dL** (5.6 mmol/L) and **125 mg/dL** (6.9 mmol/L) is classified as **pre-diabetes**. Individuals in this range are at higher risk of developing Type 2 diabetes, but their blood sugar levels are not yet high enough to be classified as diabetes.
- **Diabetes**: A fasting blood glucose level of **126 mg/dL** (7.0 mmol/L) or higher on two separate occasions confirms a diagnosis of diabetes. While the fasting blood glucose test is useful, it only gives a snapshot of an individual's blood sugar levels at a particular point in time and does not reflect how glucose levels fluctuate throughout the day. Therefore, it is often used in combination with other tests to provide a more complete picture of a person's glucose metabolism.

HbA1c Test (Glycated Hemoglobin Test)

The **HbA1c test**, also known as the **glycated hemoglobin** or **A1c test**, is one of the most widely used diagnostic tools for monitoring and diagnosing diabetes. Unlike the fasting glucose test, which only measures blood sugar at a specific time, the HbA1c test provides an **average blood sugar level** over the past **2-3 months**. Hemoglobin, a protein found in red blood cells, binds with glucose in the blood, and the HbA1c test measures the percentage of hemoglobin that has glucose attached to it.

- **Normal Range**: An HbA1c level below **5.7%** is considered normal.

- **Pre-diabetes**: An HbA1c level between **5.7% and 6.4%** suggests **pre-diabetes**. People with pre-diabetes have a higher risk of developing Type 2 diabetes.
- **Diabetes**: An HbA1c level of **6.5% or higher** on two separate occasions is used to diagnose diabetes.

One of the advantages of the HbA1c test is that it does not require fasting, making it more convenient for many individuals. However, it is important to note that certain factors, such as **anemia**, **kidney disease**, or other hemoglobin abnormalities, can affect the accuracy of the test. Additionally, the HbA1c test may not be as useful for monitoring **gestational diabetes** or for individuals with fluctuating blood glucose levels.

Oral Glucose Tolerance Test (OGTT)

The **Oral Glucose Tolerance Test (OGTT)** is another key diagnostic tool, particularly used for diagnosing **gestational diabetes** and identifying early-stage diabetes, such as **LADA** (Latent Autoimmune Diabetes in Adults). The test involves fasting overnight and then drinking a sugary solution containing **75 grams of glucose**. Blood samples are taken at intervals (usually at **1 hour** and **2 hours**) to measure how the body processes glucose over time.

- **Normal Range**: A 2-hour blood glucose level of **less than 140 mg/dL** (7.8 mmol/L) is considered normal.
- **Impaired Glucose Tolerance (IGT)**: A 2-hour blood glucose level between **140 mg/dL** (7.8 mmol/L) and **199 mg/dL** (11.0 mmol/L) is classified as **impaired glucose tolerance**, a condition often referred to as **pre-diabetes**.

- **Diabetes**: A 2-hour blood glucose level of **200 mg/dL** (11.1 mmol/L) or higher confirms a diagnosis of diabetes.

The OGTT is particularly useful for diagnosing **gestational diabetes**, as it can assess how the body's insulin response changes during pregnancy. It also helps in detecting **insulin resistance** in individuals with early Type 2 diabetes, making it a valuable diagnostic tool for identifying pre-diabetes and diabetes in its early stages.

C-Peptide Test

The **C-peptide test** measures the level of **C-peptide**, a byproduct of insulin production. When the pancreas produces insulin, it splits the insulin molecule into two parts—**insulin** and **C-peptide**—and both are released into the bloodstream. By measuring the C-peptide levels, doctors can get an indication of how much insulin the pancreas is producing. This test is particularly useful in determining whether a person has **Type 1 diabetes** (where insulin production is low or absent) or **Type 2 diabetes** (where insulin production is typically normal, but the body is resistant to its effects).

- **Low C-peptide levels** suggest that the pancreas is producing little or no insulin, which is consistent with **Type 1 diabetes** or **LADA** (Latent Autoimmune Diabetes in Adults), where insulin production declines over time.

- **Normal or high C-peptide levels** indicate that the pancreas is still producing insulin, even though the body may not be responding to it properly, which is characteristic of **Type 2 diabetes**.

C-peptide testing can also be helpful in diagnosing **insulin resistance** and monitoring how well **insulin therapy** is working in individuals with diabetes.

Role of Genetic Testing in Diagnosing Rare Types of Diabetes

While traditional blood tests are sufficient for diagnosing the more common forms of diabetes, the diagnosis of **rare types of diabetes** may require genetic testing. There are several genetic forms of diabetes, including **Maturity-Onset Diabetes of the Young (MODY), Latent Autoimmune Diabetes in Adults (LADA), Neonatal Diabetes**, and other rare monogenic forms. Genetic testing is becoming increasingly important in identifying these conditions, as they often present similarly to more common forms of diabetes but require different treatment approaches.

Maturity-Onset Diabetes of the Young (MODY)

MODY is a rare, genetically determined form of diabetes that typically presents in **young adults or adolescents**. It is caused by mutations in a single gene that affects **insulin secretion**. Because MODY often resembles **Type 1** or **Type 2 diabetes**, it can be misdiagnosed without genetic testing. There are different forms of MODY, and the most common is caused by mutations in the **HNF1A** gene, although other genetic mutations can also be responsible.

- **Genetic testing** for MODY can confirm the diagnosis by identifying specific gene mutations. This is particularly useful for differentiating MODY from Type 1 or Type 2 diabetes, as people with MODY typically do not need insulin at diagnosis and can often manage their blood sugar with oral medications.

Latent Autoimmune Diabetes in Adults (LADA)

LADA, sometimes referred to as **Type 1.5 diabetes**, is an autoimmune form of diabetes that shares characteristics of both **Type 1** and **Type 2 diabetes**. LADA typically develops in **adults over the age of 30** and is characterized by **autoimmune destruction** of insulin-producing beta cells in the pancreas, similar to Type 1 diabetes, but with a slower onset. Genetic testing can help differentiate LADA from Type 2 diabetes, as individuals with LADA have **autoantibodies** present in their blood, similar to those seen in Type 1 diabetes.

Neonatal Diabetes

Neonatal diabetes is a rare form of diabetes that affects infants under the age of **6 months**. Unlike Type 1 diabetes, which is an autoimmune disease, neonatal diabetes is caused by **genetic mutations** affecting insulin production or secretion. Genetic testing is essential for identifying the cause of neonatal diabetes, as it can help distinguish between **transient** and **permanent** forms of the disease, leading to more appropriate treatment.

Other Rare Genetic Forms

In addition to MODY, LADA, and neonatal diabetes, there are other rare genetic forms of diabetes, including **Mitochondrial Diabetes** and diabetes associated with syndromes such as **Cystic Fibrosis** or **Wolfram Syndrome**. Genetic testing plays a critical role in identifying these conditions and ensuring proper management, as the treatment approaches for these rare forms of diabetes can differ significantly from those used for Type 1 or Type 2 diabetes.

Conclusion

Diagnosing diabetes requires careful consideration of various factors, including the patient's symptoms, medical history, risk factors, and the results of diagnostic tests. **Blood tests** such as **fasting blood glucose, HbA1c**, and the **Oral Glucose Tolerance Test (OGTT)** provide valuable insights into blood sugar levels and glucose metabolism, helping healthcare professionals identify diabetes and pre-diabetes. In some cases, the **C-peptide test** may be used to differentiate between **Type 1** and **Type 2 diabetes**.

Additionally, **genetic testing** is increasingly being used to diagnose rare forms of diabetes, such as MODY, LADA, and neonatal diabetes, allowing for more precise and tailored treatment options. Early diagnosis and intervention are key to managing diabetes effectively and preventing complications, and these tests are essential tools in achieving that goal.

Chapter 14

The Role of Continuous Glucose Monitoring (CGM)

In the evolving landscape of diabetes management, **Continuous Glucose Monitoring (CGM)** has become a game-changer for both patients and healthcare providers. The ability to track glucose levels in real-time provides unprecedented insight into how the body responds to food, exercise, stress, and medications. CGMs offer a dynamic alternative to traditional methods of blood glucose monitoring, such as fingerstick tests, by providing a more comprehensive, continuous view of blood sugar fluctuations throughout the day and night.

This technology has revolutionized the way diabetes is managed, offering benefits in **glucose control**, **risk reduction**, and overall quality of life for individuals living with diabetes. However, like any technology, CGMs come with their own set of limitations and challenges, and understanding both the advantages and drawbacks of this tool is essential for making the most of it.

How Continuous Glucose Monitors (CGMs) Work

A **Continuous Glucose Monitor (CGM)** is a medical device designed to track glucose levels continuously throughout the day and night, providing real-time data that can be used to manage diabetes. Unlike traditional glucose meters, which require a fingerstick blood sample, CGMs measure glucose levels in the **interstitial fluid** (the fluid between cells) rather than directly in the blood.

Components of a CGM System

A typical CGM system consists of three main components:

- **Sensor**: The sensor is a small, flexible device that is inserted just under the skin (usually on the abdomen or arm) and continuously measures glucose levels in the interstitial fluid. The sensor is typically replaced every 7 to 14 days, depending on the brand and model.

- **Transmitter**: The transmitter is attached to the sensor and wirelessly sends the glucose data to a receiver or smartphone app. It communicates the data in real-time, updating glucose levels every few minutes.

- **Receiver/Display Device**: The receiver is the device (or smartphone app) that displays the glucose readings. Some CGMs are integrated with insulin pumps or other devices, allowing for seamless glucose monitoring and insulin delivery. The receiver shows trends, graphs, and alerts for high or low glucose levels, making it easy for users to track fluctuations.

How It Measures Glucose Levels

CGMs do not directly measure blood glucose. Instead, they measure glucose levels in the **interstitial fluid**, which reflects glucose concentrations in the blood, but with a slight delay. When a person eats, exercises, or experiences changes in their metabolism, glucose enters the bloodstream and then diffuses into the interstitial fluid. CGMs detect these fluctuations and relay the information back to the user. While the reading from a CGM may not always match the exact blood glucose value obtained by a fingerstick test, it offers an accurate and real-time view of glucose trends.

The sensor typically provides data every **5 minutes**, allowing users to see how their glucose levels are changing throughout the day and night.

These frequent updates make CGMs highly beneficial for tracking patterns and making real-time adjustments to insulin doses, meal plans, and exercise routines.

The Role of CGM in Managing Diabetes

CGMs play an essential role in improving **glycemic control**, reducing **hypoglycemia** (low blood sugar), and helping individuals make informed decisions about their daily diabetes management. This technology is beneficial for both **Type 1 diabetes** and **Type 2 diabetes**, though the specific advantages may vary depending on the type and the individual's treatment plan.

Real-time Data for Smarter Decisions

One of the most significant advantages of CGMs is the ability to track **real-time blood glucose trends**. This means that patients can receive instant feedback on how different foods, activities, medications, and stress affect their glucose levels. This continuous data stream allows individuals to:

- **Identify patterns**: By tracking glucose levels over time, users can identify patterns that indicate issues with diet, exercise, or medication regimens. For example, they may discover that certain meals cause blood sugar spikes or that exercise helps to lower glucose levels.
- **Make timely adjustments**: CGM users can make real-time adjustments to their insulin dosages, diet, or physical activity based on their current glucose levels. If glucose levels are trending upwards, users can take corrective action before they reach dangerously high levels.

- **Avoid extremes**: By having access to continuous glucose data, individuals can take steps to avoid dangerous fluctuations, such as hypoglycemia (low blood sugar) or hyperglycemia (high blood sugar), which can have serious health consequences.

Hypoglycemia Awareness and Prevention

One of the most valuable functions of a CGM system is its ability to **alert** users to dangerously low glucose levels (hypoglycemia), which is often difficult to detect in people with diabetes, especially those on **insulin therapy**. Hypoglycemia can occur suddenly and without warning, especially during sleep. CGMs can alert users when their glucose levels are trending downward, enabling them to take corrective actions before it becomes a severe issue.

These alerts are particularly important for people who experience **hypoglycemia unawareness**, a condition where individuals cannot recognize the symptoms of low blood sugar.

In addition to real-time alerts, many CGMs offer **low and high glucose thresholds** that users can customize based on their individual needs. These thresholds ensure that users are notified if their glucose levels move outside of their target range, helping them to avoid potentially dangerous situations.

Glycemic Control and HbA1c Reduction

The use of CGM has been shown to significantly improve **glycemic control** over time. Continuous glucose monitoring helps individuals keep their blood sugar levels within a tighter range, reducing the risk of both **short-term** and **long-term** complications associated with poorly controlled diabetes. Studies have shown that CGM use can lead to a **reduction in HbA1c** levels (a long-term measure of average blood sugar) without an increase in hypoglycemia. This is especially important for individuals who struggle with frequent highs and lows in blood sugar levels.

For people with **Type 1 diabetes**, where insulin therapy is required for survival, CGM technology offers a vital tool for optimizing insulin dosages and preventing dangerous episodes of **diabetic ketoacidosis (DKA)** or **hypoglycemia**.

Improved Quality of Life

For many people living with diabetes, managing blood sugar levels can feel overwhelming and time-consuming. CGMs help ease this burden by automating much of the monitoring process. Instead of performing multiple fingerstick tests throughout the day, individuals can rely on continuous glucose data. This can lead to **greater confidence** in managing diabetes and reduce the stress associated with monitoring blood sugar.

Moreover, CGMs allow users to focus on their daily life without constantly worrying about their blood glucose levels. The convenience of having a continuous stream of data at their fingertips empowers individuals to make decisions about what to eat, when to exercise, and how much insulin to administer based on their current glucose levels, rather than guessing or waiting for future symptoms.

Benefits of Continuous Glucose Monitoring

Real-Time Feedback and Trend Data

One of the key benefits of CGMs is the ability to provide **real-time feedback** on glucose levels. With continuous data, individuals can track **glucose trends** over time, identifying **patterns** and making adjustments as needed. This is particularly helpful for understanding how specific meals, activities, or medications impact glucose control.

Improved Diabetes Control

CGMs enable better **long-term blood sugar control** by providing more frequent measurements, allowing users to make more precise adjustments to their insulin doses, diet, and exercise routines. This can lead to improved **glycemic variability**, a reduction in blood sugar swings, and more stable overall glucose levels. As a result, many users experience improved **HbA1c levels** over time.

Hypoglycemia Prevention

CGMs provide an early warning system for **hypoglycemia**, helping users avoid dangerously low blood sugar levels before they cause symptoms. This ability to receive alerts for low glucose levels can be life-saving, especially during sleep when hypoglycemia may otherwise go unnoticed.

Customization and Flexibility

Most CGM systems allow for **customizable alerts** for both high and low glucose thresholds, so users can tailor the system to their specific needs and preferences. This allows people with diabetes to fine-tune their management plan and make adjustments based on lifestyle, activity levels, and other factors.

Limitations of Continuous Glucose Monitoring

While CGMs offer many advantages, there are some limitations that users should be aware of.

Cost and Accessibility

One of the primary drawbacks of CGMs is the **cost**. While the technology has become more accessible in recent years, CGMs can still be expensive, particularly for individuals without adequate insurance coverage. In addition to the cost of the device itself, there are ongoing expenses for **sensor replacements**, which need to be changed every 7-14 days, depending on the brand and model.

Accuracy and Calibration

Although CGMs are highly accurate, they are not always 100% precise. Since CGMs measure glucose levels in interstitial fluid, there can be a **lag time** of up to 15 minutes between changes in blood glucose and what the CGM sensor detects. This means that CGMs may not always reflect real-time blood sugar levels, particularly during rapid changes such as after meals or exercise. Some systems also require **calibration** with fingerstick blood glucose tests to ensure accuracy, though newer models are moving toward being calibration-free.

Sensor Adhesion and Skin Irritation

Some users experience issues with **sensor adhesion** or **skin irritation** at the insertion site. While most sensors are designed to stay in place for several days, sweating, movement, or improper placement can sometimes cause them to loosen or fall off. Additionally, some individuals may develop skin irritation or allergic reactions from the adhesive used in CGM systems.

Training and Learning Curve

Using a CGM system effectively requires a certain level of **technical knowledge** and **training**. While the technology is intuitive for many users, there may be a learning curve involved in understanding how to interpret data, set appropriate alerts, and troubleshoot issues. Additionally, some users may feel overwhelmed by the continuous flow of information and the constant monitoring of glucose levels.

Conclusion

Continuous Glucose Monitoring (CGM) has become a powerful tool for managing diabetes, offering real-time data, trend analysis, and early warning systems for glucose fluctuations. The ability to track blood sugar levels continuously throughout the day allows for **smarter decisions**, **better glucose control**, and improved **quality of life**.

While CGMs have significant benefits, including improved **hypoglycemia prevention** and **reduced glycemic variability**, they also come with limitations such as cost, accuracy issues, and the potential for skin irritation. For many individuals with diabetes, CGMs are an invaluable resource that can enhance self-management and help reduce the long-term risks of diabetes-related complications.

Chapter 15

Early Intervention Strategies

The management of diabetes, particularly Type 2 and Type 1 diabetes, requires a proactive approach, with early intervention being critical for long-term health and wellbeing. For individuals diagnosed with Type 2 diabetes, lifestyle changes made in the early stages of the disease can have a profound impact on disease progression, reducing the risk of complications and potentially even reversing or delaying the onset of full-blown diabetes.

Similarly, in Type 1 diabetes, the timing of insulin therapy is key to managing blood sugar levels effectively and avoiding long-term complications. This chapter explores the importance of early intervention strategies for both Type 2 and Type 1 diabetes, focusing on the role of **lifestyle modifications** for Type 2 diabetes and the significance of **early insulin therapy** for Type 1 diabetes.

The Importance of Early Lifestyle Modifications for Type 2 Diabetes

Type 2 diabetes is largely influenced by **lifestyle factors**, including diet, physical activity, stress, and weight management. In fact, many of the risk factors for Type 2 diabetes, such as **obesity**, **sedentary behavior**, and **poor dietary choices**, are modifiable through lifestyle changes. Early intervention in the form of **lifestyle modifications** can significantly delay or prevent the onset of Type 2 diabetes in individuals at risk, and for those already diagnosed with the condition, these changes can help **improve glycemic control**, reduce dependence on medications, and lower the risk of complications.

Dietary Changes: The Foundation of Early Intervention

The importance of a **healthy diet** cannot be overstated when it comes to preventing and managing Type 2 diabetes. In the early stages of Type 2 diabetes or pre-diabetes, **nutritional interventions** can have a significant impact on maintaining normal blood glucose levels. A diet focused on whole, minimally processed foods that emphasize **high-fiber**, **low-glycemic index carbohydrates**, and **healthy fats** can help stabilize blood sugar and reduce the body's insulin resistance.

- **Reducing refined carbohydrates**: Foods such as sugary snacks, white bread, and processed grains can cause sharp spikes in blood glucose. Replacing these with whole grains, legumes, and non-starchy vegetables can help avoid these fluctuations.
- **Emphasizing fiber**: High-fiber foods, such as vegetables, fruits, and whole grains, slow the absorption of sugar into the bloodstream, contributing to better blood sugar regulation.
- **Incorporating healthy fats**: Unsaturated fats from sources like olive oil, avocado, nuts, and fatty fish help improve insulin sensitivity and reduce inflammation, which is often elevated in Type 2 diabetes.

Dietary modifications, when made early in the course of Type 2 diabetes, can not only help manage glucose levels but may also prevent the need for more aggressive treatments, such as insulin or oral medications. In some cases, significant weight loss from diet and lifestyle changes has been shown to **reverse pre-diabetes** and even **remit Type 2 diabetes** altogether.

The Role of Physical Activity

Physical activity plays a pivotal role in both the prevention and management of Type 2 diabetes. Regular exercise improves **insulin sensitivity**, which means the body's cells become better at responding to insulin, thus helping lower blood glucose levels. Early and consistent engagement in **aerobic exercise**, such as walking, jogging, swimming, or cycling, combined with **strength training**, has been shown to enhance blood sugar control and promote weight loss, both of which are beneficial for individuals with Type 2 diabetes.

- **Aerobic exercise** helps improve cardiovascular health and aids in weight management by burning calories and increasing the body's ability to use glucose for energy.
- **Strength training** builds lean muscle mass, which increases the body's demand for glucose, further improving insulin sensitivity.

Even modest increases in physical activity, such as taking daily walks or using a stationary bike, can reduce the likelihood of developing Type 2 diabetes and can help individuals with existing Type 2 diabetes achieve better glycemic control.

Stress Management and Sleep Hygiene

Chronic stress and **poor sleep** can both negatively impact blood sugar levels by raising cortisol, a stress hormone that can lead to insulin resistance and elevated glucose levels. Early intervention through effective **stress management techniques**—such as **meditation**, **yoga**, **breathing exercises**, and **mindfulness**—can help lower stress levels, reduce blood sugar spikes, and enhance overall well-being. Moreover, prioritizing **quality sleep** is essential for improving insulin sensitivity and managing blood sugar. Consistently getting 7-9 hours of sleep per night can improve metabolic health and prevent further complications associated with diabetes.

Weight Loss and Its Impact

For individuals with Type 2 diabetes, particularly those who are overweight or obese, **weight loss** is one of the most powerful interventions. Losing even a small amount of weight—around **5-10%** of total body weight—can improve insulin sensitivity, lower blood glucose levels, and reduce the risk of long-term complications. Early weight loss interventions, such as portion control, calorie-reduced diets, and regular physical activity, can often result in significant improvements in metabolic health. For some, **bariatric surgery** has even been shown to result in **remission of Type 2 diabetes**, highlighting the powerful link between weight management and diabetes control.

How Early Insulin Therapy in Type 1 Diabetes Affects Long-Term Outcomes

While Type 1 diabetes is an autoimmune condition that results in the destruction of the insulin-producing beta cells of the pancreas, **early insulin therapy** is crucial in the management of the disease. Unlike Type 2 diabetes, where insulin resistance develops over time, Type 1 diabetes requires immediate and ongoing insulin administration for survival. The timing, **precision**, and **amount** of insulin therapy in the early stages of Type 1 diabetes can have a profound impact on both short-term and long-term outcomes, including the risk of complications and overall quality of life.

Insulin Therapy: The Foundation of Type 1 Diabetes Management

The main goal of insulin therapy in Type 1 diabetes is to mimic the body's natural insulin production as closely as possible. Early, **appropriate insulin dosing** is essential to maintain blood glucose levels within a healthy range and to avoid **hyperglycemia** (high blood sugar) or **hypoglycemia** (low blood sugar). For individuals newly diagnosed with Type 1 diabetes, the initial insulin regimen typically includes a **basal-bolus** approach, where long-acting insulin is used to cover **background insulin needs**, and rapid-acting insulin is used to cover **carbohydrates** consumed with meals.

Early Insulin Intervention and Blood Sugar Control

When insulin therapy is started promptly and correctly, individuals with Type 1 diabetes are able to avoid prolonged periods of **hyperglycemia** that can lead to the accumulation of **advanced glycation end-products (AGEs)**, which contribute to long-term complications like **nephropathy**, **neuropathy**, and **retinopathy**. Early intervention is key to maintaining normal blood glucose levels, especially in the initial months after diagnosis when blood sugar fluctuations are most extreme.

- **Good glycemic control** in the early stages of Type 1 diabetes helps reduce the risk of **diabetic ketoacidosis (DKA)**, a life-threatening condition caused by prolonged high blood sugar levels and a lack of insulin.
- **Optimal insulin management** in the first year after diagnosis has been linked to better outcomes over time, including lower rates of

microvascular complications (damage to small blood vessels), which can affect the eyes, kidneys, and nerves.

Insulin and Long-Term Outcomes: Reducing Complications

The long-term goal of insulin therapy in Type 1 diabetes is to prevent or delay the onset of **chronic complications**, such as **cardiovascular disease**, **kidney failure**, **retinal damage**, and **nerve damage**. Studies have shown that intensive insulin therapy started early in the course of Type 1 diabetes can reduce the risk of complications later in life. This is particularly evident from landmark studies like the **Diabetes Control and Complications Trial (DCCT)**, which demonstrated that strict blood sugar control in the first years of Type 1 diabetes significantly reduced the risk of complications after **30 years**.

Early insulin therapy helps to keep blood glucose levels **within a target range**, preventing the damage that can occur from **chronic hyperglycemia**. Over time, tight blood glucose control can help preserve **pancreatic beta cell function** and reduce the need for more aggressive treatment, such as insulin pumps or the introduction of other medications.

The Role of Insulin Technology

Advancements in **insulin delivery technologies**, such as **insulin pumps** and **continuous glucose monitors (CGMs)**, have further improved the management of Type 1 diabetes, especially when started early in the course of the disease. Insulin pumps deliver continuous, basal insulin and allow for precise bolus dosing around meals, while CGMs provide real-time glucose data to help fine-tune insulin doses. Early adoption of these technologies enables individuals with Type 1 diabetes to have more precise control over their blood sugar levels and reduces the burden of diabetes management.

Conclusion

Early intervention strategies are essential for managing both Type 1 and Type 2 diabetes, and can significantly improve long-term outcomes. In Type 2 diabetes, early lifestyle modifications, such as changes in diet, increased physical activity, stress management, and weight loss, can help manage glucose levels, prevent the progression of the disease, and reduce the need for medications.

In Type 1 diabetes, early and effective insulin therapy is crucial for maintaining normal blood glucose levels, preventing complications, and improving long-term health. Whether through lifestyle changes or medical interventions, the earlier diabetes is addressed, the better the chances of achieving **optimal glycemic control** and reducing the risk of complications.

Chapter 16

Medications for Diabetes

Managing diabetes involves more than just lifestyle changes; **medications** play a crucial role in controlling blood sugar levels, preventing complications, and improving quality of life for individuals with all types of diabetes. Whether it's Type 1, Type 2, or a rarer form of diabetes, pharmaceutical interventions are often necessary to complement dietary adjustments, exercise, and monitoring. In this chapter, we will explore some of the most commonly prescribed **diabetes medications**, their mechanisms of action, their side effects, and the evolving landscape of **pharmacological treatments** for diabetes.

Overview of Common Diabetes Medications

Diabetes medications are designed to lower blood glucose levels through various mechanisms, each targeting different aspects of glucose metabolism. The choice of medication often depends on the type of diabetes, the patient's individual health profile, and the specific challenges they face in managing their condition. The main classes of diabetes medications include **insulin, oral hypoglycemics,** and **injectable medications** that focus on enhancing insulin action or increasing glucose excretion.

Insulin: The Cornerstone of Type 1 Diabetes Management

For individuals with **Type 1 diabetes, insulin** is the cornerstone of treatment. Since Type 1 diabetes is characterized by the body's inability to produce insulin, external insulin is necessary to control blood glucose levels. Insulin therapy helps mimic the body's natural insulin secretion, controlling blood sugar after meals and throughout the day.

- **How Insulin Works**: Insulin lowers blood glucose by facilitating the entry of glucose into cells, where it is used for energy or stored in the liver and muscles for later use. There are different types of insulin, each with distinct properties:
  - **Rapid-acting insulin**: Works quickly to lower blood sugar after meals (e.g., insulin lispro, insulin aspart).
  - **Short-acting insulin**: Takes longer to act, but still provides post-meal blood sugar control.
  - **Intermediate-acting insulin**: Provides a steady level of insulin for about half a day.
  - **Long-acting insulin**: Helps maintain a basal level of insulin over a 24-hour period.
- **Side Effects of Insulin**: The most common side effect of insulin therapy is **hypoglycemia** (low blood sugar), which can occur if the insulin dose is too high, or if the patient skips a meal or exercises excessively. Other potential side effects include **weight gain, insulin resistance** (with long-term use), and skin reactions at the injection site.

Metformin: First-Line Treatment for Type 2 Diabetes

Metformin is the most commonly prescribed medication for **Type 2 diabetes**. It is often used as a first-line treatment because of its effectiveness, safety profile, and relatively low cost.

- **How Metformin Works**: Metformin primarily works by **reducing liver glucose production**, thereby lowering blood sugar levels. It also improves the body's sensitivity to insulin, allowing cells to take up glucose more effectively. This makes it a highly effective drug for individuals with **insulin resistance**, a hallmark of Type 2 diabetes.

- **Side Effects of Metformin**: The most common side effects of Metformin include **gastrointestinal issues** such as nausea, diarrhea, and abdominal discomfort. These symptoms often improve over time or with dose adjustments. In rare cases, Metformin can lead to a potentially life-threatening condition called **lactic acidosis**, particularly in individuals with kidney dysfunction or other contraindications.

GLP-1 Receptor Agonists: A New Class of Injectable Medications

GLP-1 receptor agonists are a relatively new class of injectable medications that have shown great promise in the management of Type 2 diabetes. These drugs work by mimicking the effects of the **glucagon-like peptide 1 (GLP-1)** hormone, which is naturally produced in the gut in response to food intake.

- **How GLP-1 Receptor Agonists Work**: GLP-1 receptor agonists help lower blood sugar by increasing insulin release in response to meals, inhibiting glucagon (a hormone that raises blood sugar), and slowing down gastric emptying. Additionally, these drugs promote satiety (feeling of fullness), which can help with weight loss—an important aspect of managing Type 2 diabetes.

- **Examples of GLP-1 Receptor Agonists**: Some common medications in this class include **liraglutide (Victoza)**, **semaglutide (Ozempic)**, and **exenatide (Byetta)**.

- **Side Effects of GLP-1 Receptor Agonists**: The most common side effects include **nausea**, **vomiting**, and **diarrhea**. These side effects typically decrease with continued use. A rare but serious side effect includes **pancreatitis**, which is inflammation of the pancreas. These medications are not recommended for people with a history of pancreatitis or certain thyroid cancers.

SGLT2 Inhibitors: Enhancing Glucose Excretion

SGLT2 inhibitors are another class of medications that have become increasingly important in the treatment of Type 2 diabetes. They work by preventing the kidneys from reabsorbing glucose, leading to increased excretion of glucose through the urine.

- **How SGLT2 Inhibitors Work**: The **sodium-glucose cotransporter-2 (SGLT2)** is a protein in the kidneys responsible for reabsorbing glucose back into the bloodstream. By inhibiting this transporter, SGLT2 inhibitors allow excess glucose to be excreted in the urine, thus lowering blood glucose levels. This class of medication also has the added benefit of promoting weight loss and lowering blood pressure, both of which are beneficial for individuals with Type 2 diabetes.

- **Examples of SGLT2 Inhibitors**: Some of the commonly prescribed drugs in this class include **canagliflozin (Invokana)**, **dapagliflozin (Farxiga)**, and **empagliflozin (Jardiance)**.

- **Side Effects of SGLT2 Inhibitors**: The most common side effects are **urinary tract infections (UTIs)**, **genital yeast infections**, and **increased urination**. In rare cases, SGLT2 inhibitors can cause **diabetic ketoacidosis (DKA)**, a serious complication in which the body produces high levels of ketones, leading to acidosis. There is also a small risk of **kidney problems** and **bone fractures** associated with these medications.

DPP-4 Inhibitors: Enhancing Insulin Response

DPP-4 inhibitors are another class of oral medications used to treat Type 2 diabetes. These drugs work by inhibiting the **DPP-4 enzyme**, which breaks down **incretin hormones**, such as **GLP-1** and **GIP**. These hormones stimulate insulin release after meals and help reduce blood sugar levels.

- **How DPP-4 Inhibitors Work**: By inhibiting the DPP-4 enzyme, these drugs increase the levels of incretin hormones in the body, which in turn enhances insulin secretion and reduces glucose production by the liver. Unlike insulin and sulfonylureas, DPP-4 inhibitors do not cause **hypoglycemia** (low blood sugar) when used alone.

- **Examples of DPP-4 Inhibitors**: Commonly prescribed drugs in this class include **sitagliptin (Januvia)**, **saxagliptin (Onglyza)**, and **linagliptin (Tradjenta)**.

- **Side Effects of DPP-4 Inhibitors**: Side effects are generally mild and may include **nasopharyngitis**, **headache**, and **stomach upset**. There is a small risk of **pancreatitis** and **joint pain** with these medications.

Sulfonylureas: Stimulating Insulin Production

Sulfonylureas are among the oldest oral medications for Type 2 diabetes. They stimulate the pancreas to release more insulin, helping to lower blood glucose levels.

- **How Sulfonylureas Work**: Sulfonylureas bind to specific receptors on pancreatic beta cells, prompting them to secrete more insulin. This can help overcome the insulin resistance often seen in Type 2 diabetes, but it does not address the underlying cause of insulin resistance.

- **Examples of Sulfonylureas**: Common examples include **glimepiride (Amaryl), glipizide (Glucotrol), and glyburide (Diabeta)**.

- **Side Effects of Sulfonylureas**: The primary side effect of sulfonylureas is **hypoglycemia**. Since they stimulate the pancreas to release insulin, they can cause a dangerous drop in blood sugar, especially if meals are missed, or the patient exercises more than usual. Weight gain is another common side effect.

The Evolving Landscape of Diabetes Medications

As research into diabetes medications continues to evolve, new treatments and combinations are being developed to better address the complexities of the disease. **Combination therapies**—where two or more medications are used together—are increasingly common, allowing for more comprehensive management of blood glucose levels. These combinations can be more effective at targeting multiple aspects of glucose metabolism, leading to better control of blood sugar with fewer side effects.

The **development of novel classes of drugs**, such as **dual GIP/GLP-1 receptor agonists** and **insulin-analog treatments**, promises even greater precision in diabetes care. These innovations aim to not only improve glycemic control but also address other health concerns commonly associated with diabetes, such as obesity, cardiovascular risk, and kidney damage.

Conclusion

Diabetes medications are a vital component of diabetes management. From **insulin** to **oral hypoglycemics**, to newer injectable treatments like **GLP-1 receptor agonists** and **SGLT2 inhibitors**, the options for controlling blood sugar levels have expanded significantly. Each medication works through a different mechanism, targeting various aspects of the body's insulin function, glucose metabolism, and organ health. While these medications can be highly effective, understanding their side effects, mechanisms of action, and appropriate use is crucial for achieving optimal outcomes in the management of diabetes.

Chapter 17

Insulin Therapy

For individuals with diabetes, **insulin therapy** is often the cornerstone of treatment. Whether for managing **Type 1 diabetes** or more advanced **Type 2 diabetes**, insulin plays a critical role in helping regulate blood sugar levels. Since diabetes, particularly **Type 1 diabetes**, is characterized by the inability to produce insulin, administering insulin from external sources is necessary to maintain blood glucose levels within a healthy range.

For individuals with **Type 2 diabetes**, insulin may be needed as the disease progresses and insulin resistance worsens. This chapter delves into the various types of insulin used in diabetes management, proper **injection techniques**, and the role of **insulin pumps** and **continuous subcutaneous insulin infusion (CSII)** systems in modern diabetes care.

Types of Insulin

Insulin is available in several different formulations, each designed to meet specific needs in blood glucose management. These insulin types differ in terms of **how quickly they act**, **how long they last**, and how they are best incorporated into a patient's treatment plan. Understanding the different **insulin types** and their functions is essential for optimizing diabetes management.

Rapid-Acting Insulin

Rapid-acting insulin is designed to begin working quickly after injection, making it ideal for controlling blood sugar spikes following meals. These types of insulin typically start to work within **15 minutes** of injection, peak around **30 to 90 minutes**, and continue to lower blood glucose for about **3 to 5 hours**.

- **How Rapid-Acting Insulin Works**: Rapid-acting insulins mimic the body's natural insulin response to food intake. They are absorbed quickly into the bloodstream and help to lower the spike in blood glucose levels that occurs after eating.
- **Examples of Rapid-Acting Insulin**: Some of the most commonly used rapid-acting insulins include **insulin lispro (Humalog)**, **insulin aspart (NovoLog)**, and **insulin glulisine (Apidra)**.
- **Usage**: Rapid-acting insulins are often injected just before meals or immediately after eating. They are used to counteract the postprandial (after meal) blood sugar rise, which is the most common challenge for people with diabetes.

Short-Acting Insulin

Short-acting insulin, also known as **regular insulin**, takes longer to begin working than rapid-acting insulin but still provides a relatively quick response. These insulins begin to work within **30 minutes** to **1 hour**, peak at around **2 to 4 hours**, and continue to act for **6 to 8 hours**.

- **How Short-Acting Insulin Works**: Short-acting insulin is typically used when insulin needs to be introduced into the bloodstream over a longer period, particularly in people who may require more stable insulin coverage during the day.
- **Examples of Short-Acting Insulin**: **Regular insulin (Humulin R, Novolin R)** is the primary short-acting insulin.

- **Usage**: This type of insulin is usually injected **30 minutes before meals** to cover the blood sugar increase that occurs after eating.

Intermediate-Acting Insulin

Intermediate-acting insulin is slower to act than rapid or short-acting insulins but provides a longer duration of coverage. It typically begins to work within **2 to 4 hours**, peaks at **4 to 12 hours**, and lasts for **12 to 18 hours**.

- **How Intermediate-Acting Insulin Works**: Intermediate-acting insulins provide a **basal level** of insulin throughout the day and night, helping to regulate blood sugar between meals and overnight.
- **Examples of Intermediate-Acting Insulin**: **NPH insulin (Humulin N, Novolin N)** is a commonly used intermediate-acting insulin.
- **Usage**: Intermediate-acting insulin is usually administered once or twice daily, often in combination with short-acting or rapid-acting insulin for meal coverage.

Long-Acting Insulin

Long-acting insulin is designed to provide a **steady, constant release** of insulin over an extended period of time, helping to maintain blood glucose control throughout the day and night without causing significant peaks or drops in blood sugar. These insulins begin to work after about **1 to 2 hours** and can last anywhere from **18 to 24 hours**, depending on the specific type used.

- **How Long-Acting Insulin Works**: Long-acting insulin mimics the basal insulin secretion of the pancreas. It helps regulate blood glucose levels between meals and overnight, providing a steady supply of insulin to meet the body's basic needs.

- **Examples of Long-Acting Insulin**: Common long-acting insulins include **insulin glargine (Lantus, Toujeo)**, **insulin detemir (Levemir)**, and **insulin degludec (Tresiba)**.

- **Usage**: Long-acting insulin is often injected once daily, though some patients may require two doses depending on their individual needs. This insulin does not cover blood sugar spikes that happen after eating, so rapid-acting or short-acting insulins are still required with meals.

Premixed Insulin

Premixed insulin combines a rapid-acting or short-acting insulin with an intermediate-acting insulin in a fixed ratio. These formulations are designed to provide both **meal-time insulin** and **basal insulin** coverage in one injection.

- **How Premixed Insulin Works**: The rapid-acting insulin portion of the premixed combination addresses the glucose spikes after meals, while the intermediate-acting insulin provides a longer-lasting basal effect to regulate blood sugar throughout the day and night.

- **Examples of Premixed Insulin**: Some examples include **Humalog Mix 75/25**, **NovoLog Mix 70/30**, and **Humulin 70/30**.

- **Usage**: Premixed insulins are typically injected **twice daily**, before breakfast and dinner, and are often preferred by patients who find it difficult to manage multiple injections or complex regimens.

Insulin Injection Techniques

Effective insulin administration requires proper technique to ensure that the insulin is absorbed correctly and works as intended. There are several methods of delivering insulin, with the most common being **subcutaneous injections** using syringes, insulin pens, or insulin pumps.

Syringes

- **How Syringes Are Used**: Traditional insulin syringes are used to inject insulin under the skin (subcutaneously). The syringe is filled with the prescribed amount of insulin, and the injection is given in the fatty tissue just under the skin, typically in the **abdomen**, **thighs**, or **upper arms**.

- **Tips for Injection**: It is essential to rotate injection sites to avoid **lipohypertrophy** (fat buildup under the skin), which can affect insulin absorption. Insulin injections should be administered with a **45- to 90-degree angle**, depending on the patient's body fat.

Insulin Pens

- **How Insulin Pens Work**: Insulin pens are pre-filled with insulin and offer a more convenient way to administer insulin compared to syringes. The dosage is adjusted using a dial on the pen, which helps individuals with diabetes more easily track and administer their insulin.

- **Advantages of Insulin Pens**: Pens are portable, easy to use, and allow for more precise dosing, making them ideal for those who need multiple injections throughout the day.

Insulin Pumps

- **How Insulin Pumps Work**: An **insulin pump** is a small, computerized device that delivers insulin continuously through a catheter placed under the skin. The pump can deliver both **basal insulin** (steady background insulin) and **bolus insulin** (for meals or corrections) throughout the day.

- **Benefits of Insulin Pumps**: Insulin pumps offer more precise control over insulin delivery and allow for **flexible dosing**. They are particularly helpful for individuals who struggle to maintain consistent blood sugar levels with injections alone.

- **Usage**: Insulin pumps require regular monitoring and adjustments to the settings, especially when food intake or activity levels change. The pump delivers rapid-acting insulin in a steady flow, and patients use a "bolus" dose to cover meals or correct high blood sugar levels.

Continuous Subcutaneous Insulin Infusion (CSII)

Continuous subcutaneous insulin infusion (CSII) is an advanced form of insulin delivery that allows for a steady, continuous infusion of insulin throughout the day. This method is typically used by individuals with **Type 1 diabetes** who require precise insulin control.

- **How CSII Works**: CSII delivers a small, continuous dose of insulin, mimicking the body's natural insulin production. Bolus doses can also be delivered via the pump to cover meals or correct blood sugar fluctuations. The pump is typically worn on the body, attached by a small tube (cannula) that injects insulin into the subcutaneous tissue.

- **Benefits of CSII**: CSII offers several advantages, including **improved blood sugar control, flexible dosing**, and the ability to adjust insulin delivery in real-time. It also reduces the number of injections required, improving comfort and convenience for the patient.

- **Challenges with CSII**: While CSII offers more precise control over insulin delivery, it requires careful management, including regular adjustments, monitoring, and troubleshooting. Additionally, it may involve higher upfront costs, and the pump requires regular maintenance, including changing the infusion site and ensuring that the insulin is properly delivered.

Conclusion

Insulin therapy is fundamental in the treatment of diabetes, particularly for those with **Type 1 diabetes** and some cases of **Type 2 diabetes**. The variety of insulin types available—ranging from **rapid-acting insulins** to **long-acting formulations**—allows healthcare providers to tailor treatment plans to an individual's specific needs.

In addition to understanding insulin types, proper administration techniques, including the use of **insulin pumps** and **continuous subcutaneous insulin infusion (CSII)** systems, are essential for optimizing diabetes management. With the right insulin regimen and consistent monitoring, individuals with diabetes can achieve better glycemic control and significantly reduce the risk of complications.

Chapter 18

Oral Medications for Type 2 Diabetes

For individuals living with **Type 2 diabetes**, managing blood glucose levels can often be achieved through a combination of lifestyle changes and **oral medications**. Unlike **Type 1 diabetes**, where insulin is the cornerstone of treatment due to the body's inability to produce insulin, **Type 2 diabetes** is primarily characterized by **insulin resistance** and the body's declining ability to use insulin effectively. As Type 2 diabetes progresses, medications become necessary to control blood sugar levels, alongside diet and exercise.

Oral medications for Type 2 diabetes work through various mechanisms to either improve insulin sensitivity, increase insulin secretion, or decrease glucose production by the liver. In this chapter, we will discuss the **different classes of oral diabetes medications**, how they function, their benefits, potential side effects, and how healthcare providers choose the appropriate medication for a patient's specific needs.

Classifications of Oral Medications

Oral diabetes medications can be broadly categorized based on their mechanism of action. While some medications primarily help the body produce more insulin, others make the body more sensitive to insulin or reduce the amount of glucose the liver produces. Here, we will explore some of the most commonly prescribed classes of oral medications.

Sulfonylureas: Increasing Insulin Production

Sulfonylureas are one of the oldest and most widely used classes of oral medications for Type 2 diabetes. These drugs work by stimulating the pancreas to release more insulin, regardless of blood sugar levels.

- **How Sulfonylureas Work**: Sulfonylureas bind to specific receptors on the pancreatic beta cells, which triggers the release of insulin. This insulin release helps lower blood glucose by allowing glucose to enter cells and be used for energy or stored for later use.

- **Commonly Prescribed Sulfonylureas**: Some of the most commonly prescribed sulfonylureas include **glimepiride (Amaryl)**, **glipizide (Glucotrol)**, and **glyburide (Diabeta)**.

- **Benefits of Sulfonylureas**: Sulfonylureas can be very effective at lowering blood sugar levels, especially in the earlier stages of Type 2 diabetes. They are often used as part of a combination therapy with other medications to achieve optimal glucose control.

- **Side Effects of Sulfonylureas**: The most significant side effect of sulfonylureas is **hypoglycemia** (low blood sugar), especially if meals are skipped, exercise is increased, or the dose is too high. Weight gain is also a common issue for individuals taking sulfonylureas, as insulin encourages fat storage. Additionally, sulfonylureas can cause **allergic reactions** or **skin rashes** in some individuals.

Biguanides: Reducing Liver Glucose Production

The most commonly prescribed **biguanide** for Type 2 diabetes is **metformin**. Metformin is typically the first-line treatment for many patients, as it is effective, has a low risk of hypoglycemia, and is relatively inexpensive.

- **How Metformin Works**: Metformin works primarily by reducing the liver's production of glucose, a process known as **gluconeogenesis**. It also improves insulin sensitivity, helping the body's cells use insulin more effectively. Additionally, Metformin can help reduce the absorption of glucose from the digestive tract.

- **Benefits of Metformin**: Metformin is well-established as the go-to medication for managing Type 2 diabetes and is typically the first medication prescribed after lifestyle changes are insufficient. It has been shown to improve long-term blood glucose control, reduce A1C levels, and, importantly, **does not cause weight gain**. Some studies also suggest that Metformin may have cardiovascular benefits, reducing the risk of heart disease, which is crucial for individuals with Type 2 diabetes who are already at higher risk.

- **Side Effects of Metformin**: While generally well-tolerated, Metformin can cause **gastrointestinal upset**, including nausea, diarrhea, and abdominal discomfort, particularly when starting the medication or adjusting the dosage. These side effects usually improve over time or with dose adjustments. In rare cases, **lactic acidosis**, a serious condition, may occur, particularly in individuals with compromised kidney function.

DPP-4 Inhibitors: Enhancing Insulin Secretion

DPP-4 inhibitors, also known as **gliptins**, represent a newer class of oral diabetes medications that work by increasing the activity of incretin hormones, which play a key role in regulating insulin secretion.

- **How DPP-4 Inhibitors Work**: Incretin hormones, such as **GLP-1** and **GIP**, are released by the gut in response to food intake and stimulate the pancreas to release insulin while inhibiting the liver from producing glucose. **DPP-4** is an enzyme that breaks down these incretin hormones, and DPP-4 inhibitors block this enzyme, thereby prolonging the effects of incretin hormones and enhancing insulin secretion after meals.

- **Commonly Prescribed DPP-4 Inhibitors**: Some of the most commonly prescribed DPP-4 inhibitors include **sitagliptin (Januvia)**, **saxagliptin (Onglyza)**, and **linagliptin (Tradjenta)**.

- **Benefits of DPP-4 Inhibitors**: DPP-4 inhibitors are generally well-tolerated and have a **low risk of hypoglycemia**. They help lower post-meal blood glucose levels and may also provide a modest reduction in A1C. These medications have a neutral effect on weight, meaning they are not likely to cause weight gain or weight loss.

- **Side Effects of DPP-4 Inhibitors**: The most common side effects are mild and include **headache**, **nasopharyngitis**, and **stomach upset**. In rare cases, DPP-4 inhibitors have been associated with an increased risk of **pancreatitis** (inflammation of the pancreas). There may also be an increased risk of **joint pain** and, less commonly, **severe allergic reactions**.

SGLT2 Inhibitors: Reducing Glucose Reabsorption

SGLT2 inhibitors represent a relatively new class of diabetes medications that work by targeting the kidneys to lower blood glucose levels. These medications not only lower blood sugar but also offer other health benefits, including weight loss and improved cardiovascular health.

- **How SGLT2 Inhibitors Work**: The kidneys play a significant role in regulating blood glucose levels by filtering and reabsorbing glucose back into the bloodstream. SGLT2 inhibitors block the **SGLT2 protein** in the kidneys, preventing glucose from being reabsorbed and instead allowing it to be excreted through urine. This reduces blood glucose levels while promoting weight loss.

- **Commonly Prescribed SGLT2 Inhibitors**: Some commonly prescribed SGLT2 inhibitors include **canagliflozin (Invokana)**, **dapagliflozin (Farxiga)**, and **empagliflozin (Jardiance)**.

- **Benefits of SGLT2 Inhibitors**: In addition to lowering blood glucose levels, SGLT2 inhibitors have been shown to provide significant **weight loss** and reduce **blood pressure**, both of which are beneficial for people with Type 2 diabetes. Furthermore, these medications have demonstrated cardiovascular and **kidney-protective** effects, reducing the risk of heart failure and chronic kidney disease, which are common complications of diabetes.

- **Side Effects of SGLT2 Inhibitors**: The most common side effects include **urinary tract infections (UTIs)**, **genital yeast infections**, and **increased urination**. In rare cases, these medications can lead to **diabetic ketoacidosis (DKA)**, a life-threatening condition. There may also be a slight increased risk of **dehydration** and **kidney problems**, so regular monitoring of kidney function is advised.

Thiazolidinediones (TZDs): Improving Insulin Sensitivity

Thiazolidinediones (TZDs), also known as **glitazones**, are another class of oral diabetes medications that work primarily by improving the body's sensitivity to insulin, especially in muscle and fat cells.

- **How TZDs Work**: TZDs activate a receptor called **PPAR-gamma** (peroxisome proliferator-activated receptor gamma), which helps cells use insulin more efficiently. By increasing insulin sensitivity, these medications reduce the body's resistance to insulin, enabling more effective glucose uptake into cells.

- **Commonly Prescribed TZDs**: The most commonly prescribed TZDs are **pioglitazone (Actos)** and **rosiglitazone (Avandia)**.

- **Benefits of TZDs**: TZDs can be effective at lowering blood glucose levels and improving insulin sensitivity, particularly in individuals with high levels of insulin resistance. These medications also offer **modest improvements in cholesterol** and **blood pressure**.

- **Side Effects of TZDs**: The most significant side effects of TZDs include **weight gain**, **fluid retention**, and an increased risk of **heart failure** in susceptible individuals. They may also increase the risk of **bone fractures** and **bladder cancer** with long-term use, though the risk is low.

How to Choose the Right Oral Medication

Choosing the right oral medication for a patient with Type 2 diabetes involves a careful consideration of several factors, including the patient's overall health, other medical conditions, lifestyle preferences, and how well they can tolerate the medication.

- **Efficacy**: Some medications may provide better blood glucose control than others. For example, **metformin** and **SGLT2 inhibitors** have demonstrated effectiveness not only in lowering blood glucose but also in improving cardiovascular and kidney health, which are key concerns in Type 2 diabetes.

- **Side Effect Profile**: Patients who are prone to **hypoglycemia** (low blood sugar) may benefit from medications like **DPP-4 inhibitors** or **SGLT2 inhibitors**, which have a low risk of causing this issue. Conversely, medications that cause **weight gain** (such as sulfonylureas and TZDs) might not be ideal for overweight individuals.

- **Coexisting Conditions**: Patients with **heart disease** may benefit from **SGLT2 inhibitors** or **GLP-1 receptor agonists**, as these medications offer additional cardiovascular protection. Those with **kidney disease** may also benefit from these drugs, as they have been shown to reduce the progression of kidney complications.

- **Cost and Convenience**: The cost of medications and their convenience in terms of dosage schedule can influence the choice of treatment. Some medications may require more frequent dosing, while others are available in once-daily formulations.

Conclusion

Oral medications for Type 2 diabetes offer a diverse range of options for individuals seeking to manage their blood sugar levels. From **sulfonylureas** that stimulate insulin secretion to **SGLT2 inhibitors** that help excrete excess glucose, each medication class offers unique benefits and potential side effects. The key to successful diabetes management is finding the right combination of medications tailored to an individual's needs, lifestyle, and health conditions. Regular follow-up with healthcare providers ensures that any adjustments to treatment can be made to optimize blood glucose control and prevent complications.

Chapter 19

Managing Hypoglycemia and Hyperglycemia

One of the primary goals in managing diabetes is maintaining stable blood sugar levels. However, fluctuations in blood sugar—both **low blood sugar (hypoglycemia)** and **high blood sugar (hyperglycemia)**—are common occurrences that individuals with diabetes must carefully monitor and manage. Understanding the causes, symptoms, and treatments for these conditions is crucial for preventing complications and improving overall diabetes control. In this chapter, we will explore the causes, symptoms, and treatments of both hypoglycemia and hyperglycemia, as well as strategies for prevention and management.

Understanding Hypoglycemia: Low Blood Sugar

Hypoglycemia refers to a condition where blood sugar levels fall below normal levels, typically defined as a blood glucose reading of **less than 70 mg/dL** (3.9 mmol/L). Low blood sugar can be a serious and sometimes life-threatening condition if not addressed quickly. It is often associated with insulin or certain oral medications that increase insulin production, but can also occur with changes in diet, exercise, or other factors.

Causes of Hypoglycemia

Hypoglycemia can occur for a variety of reasons. Some of the most common causes in individuals with diabetes include:

- **Over-medication**: Taking too much insulin or other diabetes medications that stimulate insulin release can lower blood sugar levels too much.

- **Skipping meals or snacks**: Not eating enough or skipping meals can lead to a drop in blood sugar, especially if insulin or other glucose-lowering medications are still in the bloodstream.
- **Increased physical activity**: Exercise can increase the body's sensitivity to insulin, leading to a drop in blood sugar levels if the appropriate adjustments are not made in food intake or medication.
- **Alcohol consumption**: Drinking alcohol, particularly on an empty stomach, can interfere with the liver's ability to release glucose and may lead to hypoglycemia.
- **Illness or infection**: Illnesses that cause nausea, vomiting, or a reduced appetite can interfere with the normal intake of food and lead to low blood sugar, especially if insulin doses are not adjusted.

Symptoms of Hypoglycemia

The symptoms of hypoglycemia can range from mild to severe, and it is essential for individuals with diabetes to recognize these symptoms early. Common signs include:

- **Shakiness or trembling**
- **Sweating**
- **Dizziness or lightheadedness**
- **Rapid heartbeat**
- **Hunger**
- **Irritability or mood swings**
- **Fatigue or weakness**
- **Confusion or difficulty concentrating**
- **Blurred vision**

If blood sugar continues to drop, more severe symptoms can occur, including:

- **Loss of coordination**
- **Seizures**
- **Unconsciousness**

In extreme cases, untreated hypoglycemia can lead to **coma** or death, which is why it is crucial to act quickly when symptoms appear.

Treatment for Hypoglycemia

The treatment for hypoglycemia involves quickly raising blood sugar to a safe level. The general approach is to consume fast-acting carbohydrates that can be absorbed quickly by the body. The American Diabetes Association (ADA) recommends the following:

- **15-15 Rule**: If you experience hypoglycemia, consume **15 grams of fast-acting carbohydrates** (such as glucose tablets, fruit juice, regular soda, or hard candy) and wait for **15 minutes**. Recheck your blood sugar after 15 minutes to ensure it has risen above 70 mg/dL. If your blood sugar is still low, repeat the process.

- **Avoid high-fat or high-protein foods**: These foods take longer to digest and may delay the absorption of glucose into the bloodstream.

- **Severe Hypoglycemia**: If the individual becomes unconscious or unable to swallow, **glucagon** may be administered via injection or nasal spray. Glucagon is a hormone that stimulates the liver to release stored glucose into the bloodstream.

Prevention of Hypoglycemia

Preventing hypoglycemia involves a combination of strategies:

- **Regular monitoring of blood sugar levels**: Regular testing can help detect early signs of hypoglycemia before symptoms become severe.

- **Adjusting medication**: Work with your healthcare provider to adjust medication dosages based on your activity level, meal timing, and other factors.
- **Carrying emergency supplies**: Always carry a source of fast-acting carbohydrates with you, especially when engaging in activities that may increase the risk of hypoglycemia, such as exercise or travel.
- **Eating regular meals and snacks**: Maintaining a consistent eating schedule and incorporating healthy snacks can help prevent blood sugar from dropping too low.
- **Adjusting insulin during exercise**: People with diabetes should learn how to adjust their insulin doses based on their physical activity to avoid hypoglycemia.

Understanding Hyperglycemia: High Blood Sugar

Hyperglycemia refers to elevated blood glucose levels, typically defined as a reading greater than **180 mg/dL** (10 mmol/L) after meals or **126 mg/dL** (7 mmol/L) after fasting. Unlike hypoglycemia, hyperglycemia is more common among individuals with Type 1 and Type 2 diabetes, particularly when insulin or oral medications are insufficient, or when blood sugar levels are not properly managed. It can develop gradually over hours or even days, but chronic hyperglycemia can lead to long-term complications such as **heart disease, kidney damage, nerve damage**, and **vision problems**.

Causes of Hyperglycemia

Several factors can contribute to high blood sugar levels in people with diabetes:

- **Insufficient insulin or medication**: When insulin doses are too low or oral medications are ineffective, glucose may build up in the blood.
- **Overeating**: Eating large amounts of carbohydrates or sugary foods without adjusting insulin levels can lead to elevated blood sugar levels.
- **Stress**: Emotional or physical stress can increase the release of **stress hormones** like cortisol and adrenaline, which can cause the liver to release more glucose into the bloodstream.
- **Illness or infection**: The body's response to illness or infection often leads to increased blood sugar levels as the body fights off illness.
- **Physical inactivity**: A lack of physical activity can reduce insulin sensitivity, leading to higher blood glucose levels.
- **Dehydration**: Dehydration can cause a rise in blood sugar because it reduces the volume of blood, concentrating glucose levels.

Symptoms of Hyperglycemia

The symptoms of hyperglycemia can develop slowly and may be mild at first. Common signs include:

- **Increased thirst (polydipsia)**
- **Frequent urination (polyuria)**
- **Fatigue or tiredness**
- **Blurred vision**
- **Dry mouth or skin**
- **Headaches**
- **Difficulty concentrating**

If left untreated, prolonged hyperglycemia can lead to more severe complications such as:

- **Ketoacidosis (in Type 1 diabetes)**: This condition occurs when the body starts breaking down fat for energy instead of glucose, leading to a buildup of **ketones** in the blood. If untreated, diabetic ketoacidosis (DKA) can be life-threatening.

- **Hyperosmolar Hyperglycemic State (HHS)**: This is a life-threatening complication that can occur in individuals with Type 2 diabetes, where blood glucose levels rise extremely high (often above 600 mg/dL), leading to severe dehydration and organ damage.

Treatment for Hyperglycemia

Managing hyperglycemia focuses on bringing blood glucose levels back into a safe range. Some strategies include:

- **Adjusting insulin or medication**: Individuals with Type 1 diabetes may need a correction dose of insulin to bring high blood sugar down, while people with Type 2 diabetes may need adjustments to their oral medications.

- **Exercise**: Light physical activity, such as walking, can help reduce blood sugar levels by increasing insulin sensitivity.

- **Hydration**: Drinking plenty of water helps flush excess glucose from the bloodstream through urine and helps prevent dehydration.

- **Seek medical help if necessary**: If blood sugar remains high for a prolonged period or if symptoms of **ketoacidosis** or **HHS** develop (e.g., nausea, vomiting, confusion), seek immediate medical attention.

Prevention of Hyperglycemia

Preventing hyperglycemia requires a combination of lifestyle habits, medication management, and consistent monitoring. Here are a few tips:

- **Regular blood sugar monitoring**: Regular self-monitoring of blood glucose helps detect trends that may indicate rising blood sugar levels.

- **Adherence to medication regimen**: Taking medications as prescribed and adjusting doses based on food intake and activity levels can help prevent hyperglycemia.
- **Healthy eating**: Consuming balanced meals that are rich in fiber, lean proteins, and healthy fats can prevent large spikes in blood sugar. Limiting processed foods and sugary snacks is also important.
- **Exercise**: Consistent physical activity improves insulin sensitivity and helps regulate blood sugar levels.
- **Stress management**: Learning stress-reduction techniques such as deep breathing, meditation, or yoga can help reduce the impact of stress hormones on blood sugar.
- **Stay hydrated**: Drinking enough fluids helps maintain normal blood volume and can reduce the risk of high blood sugar and dehydration.

Conclusion

Both **hypoglycemia** and **hyperglycemia** require careful management and prompt action to avoid complications. By understanding the causes, symptoms, and treatments for each, individuals with diabetes can better manage fluctuations in blood sugar levels. With appropriate prevention strategies—such as regular blood sugar monitoring, medication adjustments, healthy eating, and consistent physical activity—individuals with diabetes can minimize the risk of both high and low blood sugar, leading to better long-term health outcomes and improved quality of life. Regular communication with healthcare providers is essential for fine-tuning management strategies and making any necessary adjustments to treatment plans.

Chapter 20

The Role of Exercise in Managing Diabetes

Exercise is a cornerstone of diabetes management, playing a crucial role in improving insulin sensitivity, maintaining healthy blood sugar levels, and preventing complications associated with the disease. Regular physical activity not only helps manage blood glucose but also improves overall well-being, boosts mood, and reduces the risk of cardiovascular disease, which is heightened in individuals with diabetes. In this chapter, we'll explore the many benefits of exercise for people with diabetes, the physiological mechanisms involved, and the types of exercise that are best suited for managing the condition.

The Importance of Physical Activity for Improving Insulin

Sensitivity

One of the most significant benefits of exercise for people with diabetes is its impact on **insulin sensitivity**. Insulin sensitivity refers to how responsive the body's cells are to insulin, the hormone that helps regulate blood sugar. In people with Type 2 diabetes, **insulin resistance** occurs when the cells become less responsive to insulin, resulting in elevated blood glucose levels. Regular exercise, particularly aerobic and strength-training activities, can improve the body's ability to use insulin effectively, allowing glucose to enter cells more efficiently and reducing the amount of insulin needed to keep blood sugar levels in check.

How Exercise Improves Insulin Sensitivity

- **Increased glucose uptake by muscle cells**: During physical activity, muscles use glucose for energy, even in the absence of insulin. This helps reduce blood sugar levels and, over time, can improve the overall efficiency of insulin use. After exercise, muscles remain more sensitive to insulin for several hours, further aiding in glucose control.

- **Enhanced mitochondrial function**: Regular exercise helps increase the number and efficiency of mitochondria (the energy-producing organelles in cells). This leads to more effective energy utilization, including the use of glucose, which supports better blood sugar regulation.

- **Reduction in visceral fat**: Visceral fat (fat stored around internal organs) is a key factor in insulin resistance. Exercise helps reduce this type of fat, improving insulin sensitivity and lowering the risk of Type 2 diabetes.

- **Hormonal balance**: Exercise also triggers the release of beneficial hormones, such as **adiponectin** and **irisin**, which promote fat breakdown, improve insulin sensitivity, and help regulate blood glucose levels.

In addition to improving insulin sensitivity, regular exercise also contributes to **weight management**, which is another crucial factor in controlling diabetes, particularly for people with Type 2 diabetes. Losing even a small amount of weight can lead to significant improvements in insulin sensitivity and blood sugar control.

Types of Exercise Best Suited for People with Diabetes

While any physical activity is beneficial for people with diabetes, certain types of exercise are particularly effective in improving insulin sensitivity, blood glucose regulation, and overall health. A balanced approach that includes **aerobic exercise**, **strength training**, and

flexibility exercises is ideal for managing diabetes. Here, we will look at these different exercise modalities and their specific benefits for diabetes management.

Aerobic Exercise (Cardiovascular Exercise)

Aerobic exercise, also known as cardiovascular exercise, includes activities that increase your heart rate and improve the efficiency of your cardiovascular system. This type of exercise is highly effective for managing blood glucose levels and improving insulin sensitivity. It includes activities like walking, jogging, swimming, cycling, and dancing.

- **How it helps**: Aerobic exercise helps lower blood sugar levels during and after exercise by increasing the muscles' demand for glucose. Over time, regular aerobic exercise can enhance insulin sensitivity, reduce blood sugar fluctuations, and improve cardiovascular health, which is especially important for individuals with diabetes, who are at a higher risk of heart disease.

- **Examples of aerobic exercises**:
  - **Walking**: One of the simplest and most accessible exercises for individuals with diabetes. It can be done anywhere, requires no special equipment, and has significant benefits for blood sugar control.
  - **Cycling**: Whether on a stationary bike or outdoors, cycling helps improve cardiovascular health and aids in maintaining healthy blood sugar levels.
  - **Swimming**: A low-impact exercise that is ideal for people with joint problems or mobility issues. Swimming works both the upper

and lower body, increasing muscle strength and improving circulation.

Strength Training (Resistance Exercise)

Strength training, also called resistance exercise, involves activities that build muscle strength by working against resistance. This type of exercise is beneficial for people with diabetes because it helps increase muscle mass, improve insulin sensitivity, and enhance glucose uptake by muscle cells.

- **How it helps**: Strength training exercises promote muscle growth, which is essential for boosting metabolism and improving glucose control. Muscle tissue consumes glucose more efficiently than fat tissue, so increasing muscle mass can significantly improve insulin sensitivity and help regulate blood sugar levels.

- **Examples of strength training exercises**:
  - **Weight lifting**: Lifting free weights or using machines at a gym is an excellent way to build muscle mass and improve glucose control. For beginners, light weights with higher repetitions are recommended.
  - **Bodyweight exercises**: Push-ups, squats, lunges, and planks are great bodyweight exercises that can be done at home or in a park. These exercises engage multiple muscle groups and can be adapted to various fitness levels.
  - **Resistance bands**: Resistance bands are an inexpensive and portable way to incorporate strength training into a daily routine. They are especially useful for individuals who prefer low-impact exercise.

Flexibility and Balance Exercises

Flexibility exercises help improve joint mobility and reduce the risk of injury, while balance exercises are crucial for preventing falls, particularly in older adults with diabetes. These exercises are often overlooked in traditional fitness plans, but they are essential for overall physical health and well-being.

- **How it helps**: Improving flexibility and balance not only helps enhance movement and prevent falls, but it also contributes to better circulation and stress reduction, which can help manage blood sugar levels.

- **Examples of flexibility and balance exercises**:
  - **Yoga**: Yoga is a holistic exercise that combines flexibility, strength, and balance. It also incorporates mindfulness and deep breathing, which help reduce stress—another key factor in managing blood glucose levels. Regular yoga practice has been shown to improve insulin sensitivity, lower blood sugar levels, and reduce the risk of diabetes complications.
  - **Tai Chi**: This mind-body exercise involves slow, deliberate movements and deep breathing, promoting balance, flexibility, and relaxation. Studies have shown that Tai Chi can improve blood sugar control and reduce the risk of falls in people with diabetes.

Interval Training

High-Intensity Interval Training (HIIT) involves alternating between short bursts of intense exercise and recovery periods of lower-intensity activity. This training method has gained popularity due to its effectiveness in improving cardiovascular health, increasing endurance, and burning fat.

- **How it helps**: HIIT is highly effective in improving insulin sensitivity and reducing visceral fat. It has been shown to lower fasting blood sugar levels and improve long-term glucose control in individuals with Type 2 diabetes. HIIT workouts can also be time-efficient, providing significant health benefits in a short amount of time.
- **Examples of HIIT exercises**:
  - **Circuit training**: Alternating between strength exercises (like squats and push-ups) and aerobic exercises (like jumping jacks or sprints).
  - **Tabata workouts**: A specific form of HIIT that involves 20 seconds of all-out effort followed by 10 seconds of rest, repeated for four minutes.

The Importance of Consistency and Monitoring

While exercise offers numerous benefits for people with diabetes, it is important to maintain a consistent routine to achieve the best results. The American Diabetes Association recommends at least **150 minutes of moderate-intensity aerobic exercise per week** or **75 minutes of vigorous-intensity aerobic exercise**. Strength training should be done **two to three times per week**, while balance and flexibility exercises can be included as needed.

Before starting any exercise program, individuals with diabetes should consult with their healthcare provider, especially if they have any complications related to the heart, kidneys, or eyes. **Blood sugar monitoring** before, during, and after exercise is crucial for understanding how physical activity impacts glucose levels and adjusting insulin or medication doses as needed. It's also important to stay hydrated and wear appropriate footwear to avoid injury.

Conclusion

Exercise is a powerful tool in the management of diabetes, offering numerous benefits for both short-term and long-term blood sugar control. By improving insulin sensitivity, supporting weight management, and reducing the risk of cardiovascular disease, regular physical activity plays a vital role in optimizing health and preventing complications. A well-rounded exercise routine that includes aerobic exercise, strength training, flexibility, and balance exercises can help individuals with diabetes manage their condition more effectively and enjoy a higher quality of life. Consistency, monitoring, and tailored exercise plans are key to maximizing the benefits of physical activity in diabetes management.

Chapter 21

Nutrition and Meal Planning

One of the cornerstones of effective diabetes management is **proper nutrition**. A well-balanced diet not only helps regulate blood sugar levels but also plays a pivotal role in managing weight, improving insulin sensitivity, and reducing the risk of long-term complications associated with diabetes.

Nutrition is a tool that can significantly enhance the quality of life for individuals with diabetes, supporting both short-term blood glucose control and long-term health goals. In this chapter, we will explore the importance of **balanced meals**, **portion control**, and **carbohydrate counting**, as well as the essential role of a **registered dietitian (RD)** in helping individuals with diabetes develop personalized meal plans.

The Importance of Balanced Meals for Diabetes Management

A balanced meal is one that provides all the essential nutrients in the right proportions to meet the body's needs. For individuals with diabetes, a balanced diet helps manage blood sugar levels, supports weight management, and reduces the risk of complications like heart disease, kidney disease, and nerve damage. The primary nutrients in a balanced meal include **carbohydrates**, **proteins**, **fats**, **vitamins**, and **minerals**.

Carbohydrates: The Primary Nutrient to Watch

Carbohydrates are the primary nutrient that affects blood glucose levels, making them a key focus in diabetes management. When consumed, carbohydrates are broken down into glucose, which enters the bloodstream and raises blood sugar levels. The rate at which blood sugar rises depends on the type of carbohydrate consumed—simple carbohydrates (like sugar) are digested quickly, while complex carbohydrates (like whole grains and vegetables) are digested more slowly.

For people with diabetes, it is essential to manage **carbohydrate intake** to maintain stable blood sugar levels. This doesn't mean eliminating carbohydrates, but rather choosing healthy sources and being mindful of portion sizes.

- **Complex Carbohydrates**: Foods like whole grains (brown rice, oats, quinoa), legumes (lentils, beans), and vegetables (leafy greens, root vegetables) are rich in fiber, which helps regulate blood sugar by slowing glucose absorption. These foods also provide a wealth of vitamins and minerals, contributing to overall health.

- **Simple Carbohydrates**: Foods like candies, pastries, and sugary drinks should be limited, as they can cause rapid spikes in blood sugar. However, fruits and some dairy products, which contain natural sugars, are part of a healthy diet when consumed in appropriate portions.

Proteins: Building Blocks for Health

Proteins are essential for maintaining and repairing tissues, supporting immune function, and helping maintain muscle mass. For people with diabetes, including a variety of lean protein sources in meals is important for stabilizing blood sugar and improving satiety (feeling full).

- **Healthy Protein Sources**: These include lean meats (chicken, turkey), fish (salmon, tuna), eggs, low-fat dairy, legumes, and plant-based protein sources such as tofu, tempeh, and seitan.
- **The Role of Protein in Blood Sugar Control**: Protein does not directly raise blood sugar levels, but it can help reduce post-meal blood sugar spikes by slowing the digestion of carbohydrates. Including protein at each meal can contribute to more consistent blood glucose levels throughout the day.

Fats: The Right Fats for Heart Health

While fats are essential for overall health, it's important to choose **healthy fats** that promote heart health, as people with diabetes are at higher risk for cardiovascular diseases.

- **Healthy Fats**: Unsaturated fats, found in foods like avocados, olive oil, nuts, seeds, and fatty fish (salmon, mackerel), are heart-healthy fats that can help reduce cholesterol levels and inflammation.
- **Limiting Unhealthy Fats**: Trans fats and saturated fats, commonly found in processed and fried foods, should be limited, as they can increase the risk of cardiovascular disease and worsen insulin resistance.

Micronutrients: Supporting Overall Health

Vitamins and minerals play a vital role in maintaining overall health and well-being. People with diabetes are particularly vulnerable to certain micronutrient deficiencies, including **magnesium**, **vitamin D**, **vitamin B12**, and **potassium**.

- **Magnesium**: Found in leafy greens, nuts, seeds, and whole grains, magnesium helps regulate blood sugar and supports heart health.

- **Vitamin D**: Often low in people with diabetes, vitamin D is essential for insulin function and bone health. It can be obtained through sunlight exposure and foods like fatty fish, fortified milk, and eggs.
- **Potassium**: This mineral is important for maintaining normal blood pressure and heart function. Good sources include bananas, potatoes, beans, and leafy greens.

Portion Control: A Key to Blood Sugar Management

Portion control is a critical aspect of diabetes management. Even when eating healthy foods, consuming large portions can lead to spikes in blood sugar. Therefore, it's essential to understand appropriate portion sizes, especially when it comes to carbohydrate-rich foods.

The Plate Method

A simple and effective way to control portion sizes is using the **Plate Method**, which is a visual guide to help individuals with diabetes plan balanced meals. The method divides the plate into sections to ensure that meals are balanced:

- **Half the Plate**: Non-starchy vegetables like leafy greens, broccoli, cauliflower, peppers, or zucchini. These vegetables are low in calories and carbohydrates, making them an excellent choice for filling up without affecting blood sugar.
- **One-Quarter of the Plate**: Lean proteins like chicken, fish, tofu, or legumes. Protein helps stabilize blood sugar levels and promote satiety.
- **One-Quarter of the Plate**: Healthy carbohydrate-rich foods like whole grains (brown rice, quinoa), starchy vegetables (sweet potatoes, corn), and legumes (lentils, chickpeas). These foods provide steady energy and are rich in fiber, which helps slow glucose absorption.

Counting Carbohydrates

For many people with diabetes, **counting carbohydrates** is an effective strategy for managing blood sugar levels. Carbohydrates have the most significant impact on blood glucose, so understanding how many grams of carbohydrates are in different foods and how they affect blood sugar can help improve overall diabetes control.

- **Carb Counting Basics**: One serving of carbohydrate is generally considered to be **15 grams**. This can be found in foods like one slice of bread, half a cup of cooked rice, or a medium-sized apple. Counting carbohydrates allows people with diabetes to match their insulin doses with the amount of carbohydrates they consume, helping to avoid high or low blood sugar levels.

- **Carb-to-Insulin Ratio**: For those who use insulin, a healthcare provider may help develop a **carb-to-insulin ratio**, which specifies how many units of insulin are needed to cover a certain amount of carbohydrate intake. This ratio may need to be adjusted based on activity levels, illness, and other factors.

- **Glycemic Index (GI)**: The glycemic index is a ranking of carbohydrate-containing foods based on how quickly they raise blood sugar levels. Foods with a **low GI** (like whole grains and legumes) are digested more slowly, causing a gradual rise in blood sugar, while foods with a **high GI** (like white bread and sugary snacks) cause rapid spikes. Choosing low-GI foods can help maintain more stable blood glucose levels.

The Role of a Registered Dietitian in Meal Planning

A **registered dietitian (RD)** is a trained professional who specializes in nutrition and diet therapy. For individuals with diabetes, working with an RD can be invaluable in creating a **personalized meal plan** that aligns with individual needs, preferences, and health goals.

Benefits of Working with a Registered Dietitian

- **Personalized Meal Plans**: An RD can tailor meal plans based on an individual's age, activity level, medical history, and blood sugar patterns. They can also help with weight management goals, provide strategies for meal timing, and address cultural or dietary preferences.
- **Education on Nutrition**: RDs educate individuals with diabetes on how food choices impact blood sugar, how to read food labels, and how to incorporate healthier foods into their diet without feeling deprived.
- **Ongoing Support**: Managing diabetes through diet is an ongoing process, and an RD can provide continuous support, monitor progress, and make necessary adjustments to meal plans as needed.
- **Guidance on Supplements**: An RD can advise on the use of **vitamin and mineral supplements**, particularly for individuals with diabetes who are at risk of deficiencies in certain nutrients, like vitamin D, magnesium, or B12.

Meal Planning with a Dietitian

When working with an RD, individuals with diabetes may discuss:

- **Meal Timing**: Consistent meal timing can help regulate blood sugar levels. For some, spreading meals throughout the day and having regular snacks is beneficial to avoid large fluctuations in glucose levels.
- **Macronutrient Distribution**: A dietitian helps balance the intake of carbohydrates, proteins, and fats, tailoring the proportions of each to support optimal blood sugar control and overall health.

- **Special Diets**: For individuals with specific needs, such as those with kidney disease or cardiovascular issues, the dietitian may recommend a specialized meal plan that addresses those conditions while still managing blood sugar.

Conclusion

Proper **nutrition and meal planning** are vital components of diabetes management. A balanced diet, combined with portion control and carbohydrate counting, can help regulate blood sugar, improve insulin sensitivity, and reduce the risk of long-term complications.

By working with a **registered dietitian**, individuals with diabetes can develop personalized meal plans that meet their nutritional needs, support their health goals, and help them lead an active, fulfilling life. With the right tools, education, and support, managing diabetes through nutrition can be an empowering and effective approach to achieving optimal health.

Chapter 22

Diabetes and Mental Health

Diabetes is not just a physical condition—it profoundly impacts mental health as well. The emotional and psychological burden of managing a chronic illness like diabetes can lead to a range of mental health challenges, including **depression**, **anxiety**, and **diabetes distress**. These conditions not only affect the overall well-being of individuals with diabetes but can also interfere with their ability to manage their blood sugar and adhere to treatment plans. This chapter explores the psychological aspects of living with diabetes, the common mental health challenges associated with the condition, and effective strategies to address these challenges.

Psychological Aspects of Diabetes: The Burden of Chronic Illness

Living with diabetes can feel like a constant balancing act—monitoring blood sugar, adjusting medications, planning meals, and making lifestyle changes. This ongoing need for vigilance and self-management can lead to emotional fatigue, stress, and a sense of being overwhelmed. The mental load of managing diabetes often feels like a second job, and when emotional distress is not addressed, it can lead to poor self-care, which in turn affects blood sugar control.

Diabetes Distress: A Common Challenge

Diabetes distress is a term used to describe the emotional strain and anxiety that people with diabetes experience as they cope with the demands of managing their condition. Unlike depression or anxiety, diabetes distress is directly related to the emotional burdens of managing diabetes, and it can vary in severity. While some level of distress is common, chronic diabetes distress can interfere with a person's ability to take care of their health, leading to feelings of hopelessness, frustration, and guilt.

- **What causes diabetes distress?** Many factors contribute to diabetes distress, including the constant need for self-monitoring, the fear of complications, the frustration of fluctuating blood sugar levels, and the feeling of being judged by others for their condition. People with diabetes may also feel isolated or misunderstood by friends and family who don't fully grasp the complexities of living with the disease.

- **Symptoms of diabetes distress**: The emotional toll of diabetes distress can manifest in a variety of ways. Individuals may experience feelings of frustration, hopelessness, or exhaustion from the constant demands of managing their condition. There may be a sense of loss of control over one's health, coupled with the fear of developing complications. These feelings can make it difficult to maintain motivation and stay engaged with self-care activities like regular blood sugar testing, healthy eating, and exercise.

Depression and Diabetes: A Dangerous Combination

Depression is one of the most common mental health issues faced by people with diabetes. Research has shown that individuals with diabetes are twice as likely to experience depression compared to those without the condition. Depression can make it harder for individuals to manage their diabetes effectively, as it may diminish their energy, motivation, and ability to focus on self-care.

- **The link between depression and blood sugar control**: Depression can exacerbate the challenges of diabetes management. People with depression may struggle to keep track of their blood sugar levels, follow medication regimens, or maintain healthy eating habits. This can lead to poor blood glucose control, which in turn may worsen the symptoms of depression, creating a vicious cycle.

- **Signs of depression**: Symptoms of depression in individuals with diabetes can include persistent feelings of sadness, loss of interest in activities once enjoyed, fatigue, difficulty concentrating, changes in appetite, and sleep disturbances. If left untreated, depression can lead to significant emotional distress, a decreased quality of life, and even an increased risk of developing diabetes complications.

Anxiety and Diabetes: A Constant Worry

Anxiety is another common mental health challenge faced by people with diabetes. The uncertainty of blood sugar levels, the fear of complications, and the need to constantly monitor and adjust insulin can lead to **anxiety disorders**. In particular, individuals with diabetes may experience **generalized anxiety**, **panic attacks**, or **specific phobias** related to their health condition.

- **What causes anxiety in diabetes?** The unpredictable nature of blood sugar fluctuations, especially when they result in hypoglycemia (low blood sugar) or hyperglycemia (high blood sugar), can contribute to heightened anxiety. The fear of a severe low blood sugar episode, which can lead to confusion, fainting, or even seizures, is particularly common.

Similarly, anxiety about the long-term health consequences of poorly controlled blood sugar, such as nerve damage, kidney disease, or heart problems, can create a sense of impending doom.

- **Symptoms of anxiety**: People with diabetes who experience anxiety may exhibit physical symptoms such as rapid heartbeat, shortness of breath, sweating, dizziness, and muscle tension. Psychological symptoms may include restlessness, worry, irritability, and difficulty concentrating. The constant fear of blood sugar fluctuations and complications can lead to a heightened state of vigilance, which, over time, becomes exhausting.

Strategies to Address Mental Health Challenges in Diabetes

Addressing the mental health challenges associated with diabetes is an essential part of comprehensive diabetes care. The psychological impact of diabetes should not be overlooked, as it is intricately connected to physical health and diabetes management. Effective strategies for improving mental well-being can support individuals in managing their diabetes and improve their overall quality of life.

Psychotherapy and Counseling

Therapies such as **cognitive behavioral therapy (CBT)** and **diabetes-specific counseling** can be incredibly helpful for managing diabetes-related emotional challenges. CBT focuses on identifying and changing negative thought patterns and behaviors, making it an effective treatment for depression, anxiety, and diabetes distress. Through CBT, individuals can learn coping strategies to manage stress and develop healthier ways of thinking about their diabetes.

- **Diabetes-specific therapy**: There are also specialized counseling approaches aimed at helping people with diabetes cope with the unique challenges of managing a chronic illness. These therapies provide emotional support, encourage problem-solving skills, and help individuals set realistic goals for managing their diabetes.

Medication for Mental Health Disorders

In some cases, medication may be necessary to manage mental health issues like depression and anxiety. **Antidepressants** (such as SSRIs or SNRIs) and **anti-anxiety medications** (such as benzodiazepines or selective anxiolytics) may be prescribed by a healthcare provider to help stabilize mood and reduce feelings of anxiety. These medications can be particularly beneficial for people who are experiencing moderate to severe mental health symptoms that interfere with their ability to manage their diabetes effectively.

- **Antidepressants**: These medications work by balancing chemicals in the brain that affect mood and emotions. For individuals with diabetes, treating depression can also improve motivation and energy levels, ultimately supporting better diabetes management.

- **Anti-anxiety medications**: These medications can help manage the physical and psychological symptoms of anxiety, allowing individuals to feel more in control of their blood sugar and less overwhelmed by their health.

Stress Management and Relaxation Techniques

Managing stress is key to improving mental health in diabetes. Chronic stress can raise blood sugar levels, leading to worse blood glucose control and exacerbating both anxiety and diabetes distress.

Incorporating relaxation techniques into daily life can help individuals manage stress and improve their mental well-being.

- **Mindfulness and meditation**: Practicing mindfulness and deep-breathing exercises can reduce stress and help individuals feel more in control of their emotions. These techniques have been shown to lower cortisol levels, reduce anxiety, and improve blood glucose control.
- **Yoga and physical activity**: Physical activity is a powerful stress reliever. Regular exercise, particularly activities like yoga, which combine movement with mindfulness, can help lower stress, improve mood, and enhance insulin sensitivity.

Support Systems and Peer Support

Having a strong support network is essential for mental health in diabetes. Support from family, friends, and healthcare providers can make a huge difference in how individuals cope with the challenges of managing diabetes. Peer support, such as diabetes support groups or online forums, can provide a sense of community and understanding from others who are going through similar experiences.

- **Support groups**: Group settings, whether in-person or online, allow individuals to share their experiences, learn from others, and receive encouragement. These groups can provide a sense of validation and help individuals realize they are not alone in their struggles.
- **Family involvement**: Educating family members about the emotional challenges of diabetes and how they can provide support is crucial. Encouragement from loved ones can reduce feelings of isolation and frustration, and having a strong support system can promote adherence to treatment plans and improve mental health outcomes.

Education and Self-Management

One of the most effective ways to reduce anxiety and diabetes distress is through **education and self-management**. Knowledge about diabetes, its management, and the potential complications can help individuals feel more empowered and in control of their condition. Structured education programs, like those provided by diabetes educators or in diabetes self-management courses, can teach people how to manage their blood sugar, make healthier lifestyle choices, and cope with the emotional demands of diabetes.

- **Diabetes self-management programs**: These programs provide individuals with the tools they need to make informed decisions about their diabetes care. They can also include components that address mental health, such as strategies for managing stress and improving emotional well-being.

Conclusion

The psychological aspects of living with diabetes are significant and should not be underestimated. **Diabetes distress, depression**, and **anxiety** are common challenges that can hinder diabetes management and impact overall quality of life. However, with the right support, education, and treatment, these mental health challenges can be addressed. Whether through psychotherapy, medication, stress management, or the support of family and peers, individuals with diabetes can develop effective strategies to cope with the emotional toll of the disease. By addressing both the physical and emotional aspects of diabetes, people with the condition can lead healthier, more fulfilling lives.

Chapter 23

Building a Diabetes-Friendly Lifestyle

Living with diabetes requires an ongoing commitment to maintaining healthy habits and making thoughtful lifestyle choices that support both physical and mental well-being. While diabetes management can seem overwhelming at times, creating a **diabetes-friendly lifestyle** doesn't mean that the condition has to define or control every aspect of life. It's about integrating health-promoting habits into daily routines in a way that feels manageable and sustainable, allowing individuals to thrive without letting diabetes take over. In this chapter, we will explore how to build a balanced, fulfilling lifestyle that supports diabetes management, promotes overall wellness, and enables people to live life to its fullest.

Creating Daily Routines that Promote Health and Wellness

A structured daily routine is one of the most powerful tools in managing diabetes effectively. **Consistency** is key when it comes to controlling blood sugar levels, improving insulin sensitivity, and reducing the risk of complications. By developing routines that prioritize both physical and mental health, individuals with diabetes can ensure that they are proactively managing their condition, while also maintaining balance and quality of life.

Morning Routines for a Healthy Start

The way the day starts sets the tone for how well individuals can manage their diabetes throughout the day. Establishing a **morning**

routine that focuses on health can help set a positive mindset and create a sense of control over blood sugar levels.

- **Blood sugar monitoring**: For many individuals with diabetes, checking blood glucose first thing in the morning is a crucial part of the daily routine. This helps to understand overnight glucose trends and make adjustments to diet, exercise, or medication as needed. **Fasting blood sugar** levels are particularly important to track, as high morning readings may indicate inadequate overnight insulin levels or the dawn phenomenon, where blood sugar spikes early in the morning due to hormonal fluctuations.

- **Healthy breakfast**: A balanced breakfast is essential to help start the day with stable blood sugar. **Whole grains** like oats or quinoa, along with **protein** from sources like eggs or Greek yogurt, and **healthy fats** from avocado or nuts, can provide steady energy and support blood sugar control. A breakfast that includes fiber-rich foods will also help prevent a post-meal glucose spike.

- **Hydration**: Drinking water is vital for hydration, as it helps maintain kidney function and flushes out excess sugar in the urine. Avoid sugary drinks, which can cause spikes in blood glucose. Starting the day with a glass of water can help rehydrate the body after a night's sleep.

Midday and Evening Routines to Stay on Track

While mornings are important for setting a strong foundation, the rest of the day requires mindful attention to ensure consistent blood sugar control. Establishing healthy **midday and evening routines** can make it easier to manage diabetes while continuing with work, family, and social activities.

- **Meal planning and portion control**: Creating and sticking to a **meal plan** can reduce the likelihood of impulsive eating and unhealthy choices. Planning meals in advance allows for **portion control**, helping to balance the intake of **carbohydrates**, **proteins**, and **fats** at each meal. Avoiding large, carb-heavy meals can prevent blood sugar spikes.

- **Exercise routine**: Regular physical activity is crucial for improving insulin sensitivity, managing weight, and reducing stress. Scheduling exercise into the daily routine makes it easier to stay committed. Exercise doesn't have to be overly strenuous—**moderate activities** such as walking, swimming, or yoga can be highly effective in managing blood glucose. It's also important to note that exercise has immediate benefits for blood sugar control, helping muscles absorb glucose more efficiently.

- **Meal timing**: Spacing meals throughout the day and eating at regular intervals is essential for maintaining blood sugar levels within the desired range. Eating smaller, more frequent meals helps avoid overeating and supports steady energy levels. Many people with diabetes find it beneficial to have **snacks** between meals, especially when they're on insulin, to prevent dips in blood sugar levels.

- **Mindful eating**: Being aware of how food affects blood sugar can empower individuals with diabetes to make informed choices. Paying attention to hunger cues, savoring meals, and eating slowly can improve digestion, help with portion control, and prevent overeating.

Evening Wind-Down for Restful Sleep

Getting quality **sleep** is essential for managing diabetes effectively. Poor sleep can disrupt blood sugar regulation and increase insulin resistance. Therefore, establishing an evening routine that prioritizes rest is crucial for overall health and wellness.

- **Avoiding late-night snacks**: Eating too close to bedtime can raise blood sugar levels, particularly if the snack is high in carbohydrates or sugar. If a snack is necessary before bed, choose **protein-based snacks** such as a handful of nuts or a small serving of cottage cheese, which have a minimal impact on blood sugar.

- **Relaxation techniques**: Stress can have a negative impact on blood sugar, so incorporating relaxation techniques before bed can help to lower cortisol levels and promote better sleep. Practices like **deep breathing**, **progressive muscle relaxation**, or even **light stretching** can help calm the mind and body, ensuring a restful night's sleep.

- **Consistent sleep schedule**: Going to bed and waking up at the same time every day helps regulate the body's internal clock and supports better sleep quality. A good night's sleep can enhance insulin sensitivity, improve energy levels, and contribute to a more balanced emotional state.

How to Make Diabetes a Part of Everyday Life Without Letting It Take Over

While diabetes management requires ongoing attention, it should not dominate every aspect of life. The goal is to integrate diabetes care seamlessly into daily routines without letting it become overwhelming. Here are a few strategies to help individuals live life to the fullest while keeping diabetes in check:

Empowering Yourself with Knowledge

Understanding the intricacies of diabetes empowers individuals to make informed decisions about their health. By educating oneself about diabetes management, blood sugar fluctuations, medications, and the impact of lifestyle choices, individuals can feel more confident in their ability to manage the disease. This sense of control reduces the emotional burden of diabetes and helps people incorporate health habits into daily life with greater ease.

Finding Support and Building Connections

Social support plays a key role in successfully managing diabetes. Whether through family, friends, or **support groups**, connecting with others who understand the challenges of living with diabetes can provide emotional encouragement and practical tips for day-to-day management. Engaging with a community of people with diabetes can help reduce feelings of isolation and remind individuals that they are not alone in their journey.

- **Online communities** and **peer support groups** offer an opportunity for individuals to share their experiences, ask questions, and receive guidance from others who are facing similar challenges. Additionally, support from healthcare providers such as **diabetes educators**, **dietitians**, and **counselors** can provide expert advice and help individuals tailor their diabetes management plan to fit their lifestyle.

Setting Realistic Goals and Expectations

It's important to set **realistic goals** when it comes to diabetes management. While striving for optimal blood glucose control is essential, expecting perfection can create undue stress and frustration.

Instead, focus on making gradual, sustainable changes that fit into daily life. Celebrate small victories, such as consistent blood sugar monitoring, sticking to a healthy meal plan, or completing a daily walk.

- **Long-term success** comes from developing a mindset of **progress** rather than perfection. Understanding that there will be challenges along the way—and that it's okay to have setbacks—can help individuals stay motivated and resilient.

Making Room for Fun and Flexibility

It's essential to make time for activities that bring joy and relaxation, whether that's spending time with loved ones, pursuing hobbies, or engaging in outdoor activities. Diabetes management doesn't mean sacrificing the things that make life enjoyable. With careful planning and flexibility, it is possible to enjoy special occasions, dine out, or travel while still taking good care of one's health.

- **Flexibility** in managing diabetes can make the condition feel less restrictive. For example, if an individual wants to indulge in a favorite treat, they can plan ahead by adjusting their insulin or meal plan to accommodate that choice. The key is to enjoy life without feeling like diabetes has to dictate every decision.

Conclusion

Building a **diabetes-friendly lifestyle** involves creating daily routines that prioritize **health and wellness** while allowing individuals to thrive in all aspects of life. By focusing on **healthy habits**, managing stress, and integrating diabetes management into everyday activities, individuals can maintain control of their condition without letting it take over their lives. Embracing diabetes as part of daily life—rather than allowing it to dominate—helps create a balanced, fulfilling life that includes both the necessary care and the freedom to enjoy all that life has to offer. The journey with diabetes may require ongoing adjustments, but with the right mindset, support, and strategies, it's possible to live a vibrant, rewarding life.

Chapter 24

Managing Diabetes While Traveling

Traveling can be an exciting and rewarding experience, but for individuals with diabetes, it often requires extra preparation and vigilance. Whether it's a weekend getaway or an international vacation, managing blood sugar levels, maintaining medication schedules, and navigating unfamiliar environments can pose unique challenges. However, with the right strategies in place, people with diabetes can enjoy their travels without compromising their health. In this chapter, we will explore essential tips for managing blood sugar levels while traveling, as well as the role of **health passports** and **travel documentation** in ensuring a smooth journey.

Tips for Managing Blood Sugar Levels While Traveling

Traveling often involves changes in routine, including altered meal schedules, changes in physical activity levels, new foods, and different time zones. These disruptions can affect blood sugar levels, making it essential to plan ahead to prevent complications. Here are several key tips for managing diabetes effectively while traveling:

Prepare and Plan Ahead

The first step to managing diabetes while traveling is **preparation**. Having a clear plan ensures that you can address any potential issues that may arise during your trip. Some important steps to take when preparing for travel include:

- **Consulting your healthcare provider**: Before embarking on any trip, it's a good idea to meet with your healthcare provider, particularly if you are traveling internationally or will be in an unfamiliar environment. Your doctor can provide advice on managing blood sugar levels, adjusting medications for time zone changes, and specific recommendations for the type of travel you're planning.

- **Organizing supplies**: Make sure you pack all the necessary **medications** (insulin, oral diabetes medications, blood sugar test strips, etc.) in sufficient quantities to cover the entire trip, with extra in case of delays or unforeseen circumstances. This includes **syringes**, **pens**, or **insulin pumps**, as well as **glucose monitoring devices**. Carrying supplies in both your carry-on and checked luggage ensures you always have access to your diabetes management tools.

- **Researching destination specifics**: If you're traveling abroad, research the availability of healthcare services, insulin, and other diabetes-related supplies in the area. It's also wise to learn about the local food culture, as well as the typical meal schedules, to better plan your diet while away.

Time Zone Adjustments and Medication Scheduling

One of the most significant challenges for travelers with diabetes is adjusting to new **time zones**, particularly if you take insulin or other medications that need to be administered at specific times. Shifting your medication schedule gradually before your trip can help your body adjust more smoothly to the time zone change.

- **Adjusting insulin timing**: If you are traveling across multiple time zones, consider how your **insulin injections** or **insulin pump schedules** might need to be altered. Work with your healthcare provider to adjust the timing of your doses to match your destination's time zone.

- **Taking medications with you**: Always bring medications in their original packaging, along with the prescription or a note from your doctor, in case you need to refill or verify your medications while abroad. In some countries, certain medications might not be available or might require special authorization, so planning ahead is crucial.

Maintaining Consistent Blood Sugar Monitoring

Maintaining regular blood sugar monitoring while traveling is essential, particularly since **meal timing**, **activity levels**, and **stress** from travel can cause fluctuations in glucose levels. Whether you are managing your blood sugar with **insulin** or oral medications, frequent testing is important to ensure that your levels stay within a safe range.

- **Carrying a portable glucose meter**: Always have a **blood glucose meter** with you, along with extra test strips and lancets. Having this equipment easily accessible will allow you to check your levels before meals, during periods of physical activity, and if you feel unwell or experience symptoms of high or low blood sugar.

- **Using continuous glucose monitoring (CGM)**: If you use a **CGM system**, this can be an especially helpful tool for managing diabetes while traveling. Continuous monitoring will give you real-time feedback on your glucose levels, allowing you to take immediate action if necessary. Be sure to pack extra sensors and ensure that you have a reliable power source for the receiver or smartphone app that tracks the data.

Managing Meals and Snacks

Maintaining a balanced diet is another key component of managing blood sugar levels while traveling. The excitement of being in a new place can lead to indulging in unfamiliar foods or eating on the go, which may disrupt your blood sugar control. Here are some tips for managing your meals:

- **Planning meals and snacks**: Research local cuisine and **meal times** before your trip. Having a plan for when and what you will eat helps prevent overeating or consuming too many carbohydrates in a single sitting. Always carry **healthy snacks**—like nuts, fruit, or protein bars—if you're unsure about meal availability during long periods of travel, such as during flights or bus rides.

- **Portion control**: Many restaurants and food vendors in different countries serve large portions. Pay attention to portion sizes and try to **balance meals** by incorporating lean proteins, whole grains, and non-starchy vegetables. You can also ask for modifications, like dressing on the side or substituting starchy sides with extra vegetables.

- **Avoiding sugary drinks**: When traveling, it's easy to be tempted by sugary drinks or juices, especially if they're part of the local culture. Choose **water** or **unsweetened beverages** instead. If you need to drink something sweet, try to manage your intake by choosing low-calorie or sugar-free options, or have a small serving and balance it with other meals.

Staying Active and Managing Stress

Physical activity plays a significant role in diabetes management by improving **insulin sensitivity**, stabilizing blood sugar, and reducing stress. Traveling provides opportunities to engage in **active sightseeing** or outdoor adventures that can contribute to your overall health.

- **Walking and exploring**: Consider incorporating **walking tours**, hiking, or other physical activities into your daily itinerary. Not only does exercise help with blood sugar control, but it also helps reduce travel stress and improve sleep quality.

- **Maintaining your routine**: If you're used to a regular exercise routine, try to maintain it while on vacation. Whether it's a morning yoga session, a swim in the hotel pool, or a jog in the local park, staying active will help you feel better physically and mentally.

- **Stress management**: Traveling can sometimes be stressful, especially if unexpected delays or issues arise. Practice relaxation techniques like **deep breathing**, **meditation**, or **progressive muscle relaxation** to manage any anxiety or stress. Reducing stress helps keep blood sugar levels more stable and prevents emotional eating.

The Role of Health Passports and Travel Documentation for People with Diabetes

Traveling with diabetes requires careful documentation to ensure that you are prepared for emergencies, have access to necessary medical care, and can easily communicate your condition to healthcare providers when needed. **Health passports** and other travel documentation are invaluable tools that help provide peace of mind while traveling.

Health Passport: A Key Travel Document

A **health passport** is a comprehensive document that includes essential health information for travelers with chronic conditions like diabetes. Having a health passport ensures that your medical needs are clearly communicated, particularly in foreign countries where there may be language barriers or differences in medical practices.

- **What to include in a health passport**: Your health passport should contain detailed information about your diabetes, including your diagnosis, treatment plan, and medications. Be sure to include contact information for your healthcare provider, a list of your medications (with dosages), and any allergies you may have. It's also helpful to include emergency instructions, such as what to do if you experience hypoglycemia or hyperglycemia.

- **Language considerations**: If you're traveling abroad, it's a good idea to have your health passport translated into the local language to make it easier for local healthcare providers to understand your needs. Some health passports even offer multilingual translation for key medical phrases.

Other Important Travel Documentation

In addition to a health passport, there are other important documents and considerations to keep in mind when traveling with diabetes:

- **Doctor's note**: Carry a **letter** from your healthcare provider outlining your diabetes diagnosis and medication regimen. This letter can be especially helpful when passing through airport security or if you need medical attention during your trip.

- **Travel insurance**: Ensure that your **travel insurance** covers **chronic conditions** like diabetes, including emergency medical treatment for diabetes-related complications. Some insurance providers offer specific coverage for medical conditions, so it's worth reviewing the policy details before booking your trip.

- **Medication and supplies documentation**: Keep copies of your **prescriptions** and medication packaging to avoid issues at customs or pharmacies while traveling. In some countries, importing certain medications may require special permits, so be sure to check the rules of your destination country before you travel.

Conclusion

Traveling with diabetes may require a bit more planning and preparation, but with the right strategies and tools, it's possible to enjoy new experiences and explore the world without compromising your health. By staying on top of blood sugar monitoring, meal planning, physical activity, and carrying the necessary travel documentation, individuals with diabetes can manage their condition with confidence.

A **health passport** and proper **documentation** can further ease the process, ensuring that you have access to the right care if needed. With careful planning, travel can be an enriching experience that enhances your life, providing lasting memories while supporting your health and well-being.

Chapter 25

Diabetes and Aging

As individuals age, the body undergoes numerous physiological changes that can affect overall health and well-being. For older adults with diabetes, these age-related changes can present unique challenges in managing the condition. Diabetes in the elderly is not just about managing blood sugar levels—it's also about navigating complex interactions between medications, other chronic conditions, cognitive health, and lifestyle factors. Understanding how diabetes affects aging adults differently, and employing tailored strategies for management, is crucial for ensuring a better quality of life and reducing the risk of complications. In this chapter, we'll explore how diabetes impacts older adults, and discuss practical strategies for managing the disease in this population.

How Diabetes Affects Older Adults Differently

Diabetes in older adults often presents with additional complexities compared to younger individuals. Age-related changes in metabolism, organ function, and muscle mass can influence the progression and management of diabetes, requiring special attention and a personalized approach.

Changes in Insulin Sensitivity and Metabolism

As people age, their body's ability to process and utilize insulin typically declines. **Insulin resistance**, a hallmark of Type 2 diabetes, often worsens with age. Older adults tend to have less muscle mass, which reduces the body's ability to use glucose efficiently. Additionally,

fat distribution changes with age, leading to increased abdominal fat, which has been linked to increased insulin resistance.

Along with changes in insulin sensitivity, the pancreas's ability to produce insulin may also decrease over time. This can make it more challenging for older adults to maintain normal blood sugar levels, especially if they have Type 2 diabetes. In some cases, the pancreas may not produce enough insulin, even though the body is resistant to its effects. This can make blood sugar management more difficult and can lead to **fluctuations** in blood glucose.

Impaired Kidney Function

As people age, **kidney function** naturally declines, and this can impact the way the body handles both glucose and insulin. In individuals with diabetes, kidney damage is a common complication that can worsen with age. High blood sugar levels over time can cause damage to the blood vessels in the kidneys, leading to diabetic nephropathy. Kidney damage in the elderly may also reduce the body's ability to excrete excess glucose, which can lead to higher blood sugar levels. Additionally, certain diabetes medications, especially those excreted through the kidneys, may need to be adjusted as kidney function decreases.

Increased Risk of Cardiovascular Disease

Older adults with diabetes are at a significantly higher risk for **cardiovascular diseases**, including heart attacks, strokes, and peripheral artery disease. Diabetes accelerates the aging process of the blood vessels, causing **atherosclerosis**, or the thickening and hardening of the arteries, which can lead to reduced blood flow to vital organs and tissues.

Older adults with diabetes often have multiple risk factors for heart disease, including high blood pressure, high cholesterol, and obesity, all of which can complicate blood sugar management and increase the risk of heart-related complications.

Cognitive Decline and Diabetes

The impact of diabetes on cognitive health is another concern for older adults. Research suggests that people with diabetes, particularly those with poorly controlled blood sugar levels, are at an increased risk for **dementia** and **cognitive decline**. High blood glucose levels may contribute to changes in the brain that lead to memory loss, confusion, and difficulty concentrating. In addition, some diabetes medications can have side effects that exacerbate cognitive issues, making it important to regularly assess cognitive function in elderly individuals with diabetes.

Strategies to Manage Diabetes in Older Populations

Managing diabetes in older adults requires a comprehensive approach that addresses the unique challenges of aging while balancing the need for effective blood sugar control. The following strategies can help older adults with diabetes optimize their health, reduce complications, and maintain a high quality of life.

1. Tailored Medication Management

Medication management for older adults with diabetes must take into account both the individual's **health status** and their **cognitive function**. Many elderly people are on multiple medications to manage comorbidities such as hypertension, high cholesterol, and arthritis, which can complicate diabetes management.

- **Medication simplification**: Polypharmacy (the use of multiple medications) is a common concern among older adults. The more medications an individual takes, the higher the risk of **drug interactions** and medication errors. Healthcare providers should aim to simplify the medication regimen whenever possible, focusing on medications that are most effective and suitable for the patient's individual health needs.

- **Insulin management**: For some older adults with diabetes, insulin therapy may need to be adjusted to account for changes in insulin sensitivity, kidney function, and potential cognitive impairments. Long-acting insulin or **insulin pumps** may be more practical for elderly individuals who have difficulty managing multiple injections. It's also important to adjust insulin doses based on meal timing, physical activity, and blood glucose levels to avoid episodes of **hypoglycemia** (low blood sugar), which can be particularly dangerous for older adults.

- **Oral medications**: **Metformin**, **sulfonylureas**, and **GLP-1 receptor agonists** are common oral medications used to treat Type 2 diabetes in the elderly. However, these medications need to be carefully monitored for potential side effects, especially in those with kidney impairment. **SGLT2 inhibitors** are increasingly used, but they can be associated with increased risks of dehydration and urinary tract infections, so careful monitoring is required.

2. Blood Sugar Monitoring and Regular Check-Ups

Older adults may experience **variation in blood sugar levels** due to changes in lifestyle, diet, medication, and comorbid conditions. Regular blood sugar monitoring is essential to ensure that levels remain within the target range and to detect any early signs of complications.

- **Frequent blood glucose checks**: Monitoring blood sugar frequently, especially before meals and before bedtime, can help detect patterns in blood glucose fluctuations. This is particularly important in the elderly, who may have reduced sensation or **hypoglycemia unawareness** (a condition where they cannot feel the symptoms of low blood sugar).

- **A1c target goals**: For older adults, the ideal A1c target may be slightly higher than for younger individuals, depending on their overall health and life expectancy. For many older adults, especially those with multiple comorbid conditions or frailty, a more relaxed A1c goal of around 7.5%–8% may be appropriate. However, individual goals should always be discussed with a healthcare provider.

3. Nutritional Support and Meal Planning

Diet plays a critical role in managing diabetes, especially for older adults, who may face additional challenges such as **loss of appetite**, **dental issues**, or difficulty preparing meals. A well-balanced, diabetic-friendly diet can help control blood sugar, manage weight, and improve overall health.

- **Carbohydrate control**: Older adults with diabetes should focus on a diet that includes **complex carbohydrates**—such as whole grains, vegetables, and legumes—while limiting **simple sugars** and highly processed foods. **Carbohydrate counting** can help manage blood glucose levels by ensuring that meals provide a steady supply of energy without causing spikes in blood sugar.

- **Balanced meals**: Incorporating lean proteins, healthy fats, and fiber-rich foods can help manage hunger and prevent blood sugar fluctuations. Working with a **registered dietitian** can help older adults develop a personalized meal plan that accounts for their individual preferences, cultural background, and any other medical conditions.

- **Hydration**: Older adults with diabetes are at an increased risk of dehydration, particularly if they have **kidney disease** or are taking medications that increase urination (like **SGLT2 inhibitors**). It's essential to maintain adequate hydration, as dehydration can affect blood sugar regulation and kidney function.

4. Physical Activity and Mobility

Exercise is one of the most effective ways to manage Type 2 diabetes, and it offers a wide range of health benefits, particularly for older adults. However, physical activity needs to be adapted to the individual's physical capabilities and health status.

- **Exercise goals**: Older adults should aim for at least **150 minutes of moderate-intensity aerobic activity** each week, such as walking, swimming, or cycling. Strength training exercises can also help maintain muscle mass and improve insulin sensitivity, which naturally declines with age. Even small amounts of activity, such as walking after meals, can significantly help in managing blood sugar.

- **Physical therapy**: For older adults with mobility issues, working with a **physical therapist** can help develop a safe and effective exercise plan that accommodates physical limitations while still providing health benefits.

5. Managing Comorbid Conditions

Older adults with diabetes are often managing several other health conditions simultaneously. Conditions like **hypertension, arthritis, hearing loss**, and **vision problems** can affect diabetes management and overall quality of life. A holistic approach to care is necessary to address these comorbidities and prevent complications.

- **Regular check-ups**: In addition to blood sugar monitoring, older adults with diabetes should have regular screenings for other chronic conditions, such as heart disease, kidney function, and eye health. Early detection and management of comorbidities can prevent more severe complications down the road.

- **Mental health support**: Depression and **diabetes distress** are common in older adults, and these psychological factors can impact blood sugar management. Mental health support, including counseling or **therapy**, is crucial for improving both emotional well-being and diabetes control.

Conclusion

Managing diabetes in older adults requires a comprehensive, individualized approach that considers the unique challenges associated with aging. By addressing changes in **insulin sensitivity**, **kidney function**, and **cognitive health**, healthcare providers and individuals can work together to optimize diabetes management and prevent complications.

Tailoring medication regimens, monitoring blood sugar regularly, focusing on balanced nutrition, maintaining physical activity, and managing comorbidities are all essential elements of a successful diabetes care plan for older adults. With the right strategies, older adults with diabetes can lead healthy, fulfilling lives and enjoy their later years with confidence and vitality.

Chapter 26

Diabetes and Pregnancy

Pregnancy is a transformative and often joyous time in a woman's life, but for those living with diabetes, it comes with unique challenges. Both pre-existing diabetes (Type 1 or Type 2) and gestational diabetes (GDM) require careful management to ensure the health and safety of both the mother and her baby. Blood sugar levels that are too high or too low can lead to complications during pregnancy and delivery, making careful monitoring and timely intervention essential. This chapter delves into how diabetes affects pregnancy, how to manage the condition before, during, and after pregnancy, and the risks and special considerations for pregnant women with diabetes.

Managing Diabetes Before Pregnancy

Managing diabetes before pregnancy is crucial for both the woman's health and the health of her future child. Proper blood glucose control can reduce the risk of pregnancy complications, such as **miscarriage**, **birth defects**, and **preterm birth**.

Optimizing Blood Sugar Control

The primary goal for women with diabetes who are planning to become pregnant is to optimize **blood glucose control** before conception. This often involves working closely with a healthcare team, including an obstetrician, endocrinologist, and registered dietitian, to ensure that blood sugar levels are within a healthy range. Women with diabetes should aim for an **A1c** level below 6.5% before pregnancy. This level minimizes the risk of **birth defects** and other complications associated with poorly controlled blood sugar.

Blood sugar fluctuations—whether from **hyperglycemia** (high blood sugar) or **hypoglycemia** (low blood sugar)—can have long-lasting effects on both maternal and fetal health. Therefore, women should focus on achieving stable glucose control with appropriate lifestyle changes and medications.

Preconception Counseling

Preconception counseling is critical for women with diabetes to discuss potential risks and create a management plan tailored to their health needs. Key components of preconception counseling include:

- **Reviewing medication use**: Some medications used to manage diabetes (such as **ACE inhibitors** and **statins**) are not recommended during pregnancy. A healthcare provider will review current medications and switch to pregnancy-safe alternatives, such as **insulin** or **metformin**, as appropriate.

- **Nutritional planning**: Women should work with a dietitian to create a balanced eating plan that supports pregnancy while keeping blood sugar levels stable. A focus on **low glycemic index foods, fiber, lean proteins**, and healthy fats is essential for managing blood glucose levels.

- **Physical activity**: Regular physical activity is important for improving insulin sensitivity and maintaining a healthy weight before pregnancy. However, certain types of exercise may need to be modified depending on a woman's overall health and fitness level.

Managing Other Health Conditions

Pregnant women with diabetes often have other health conditions that require attention, such as **hypertension**, **hyperlipidemia**, or **obesity**. It is essential to manage these conditions prior to pregnancy to reduce the risk of complications during pregnancy and childbirth. Regular screenings for **diabetic retinopathy**, **kidney function**, and **nerve damage** should be done to ensure that diabetes-related complications do not affect the pregnancy.

Managing Diabetes During Pregnancy

Pregnancy places significant demands on a woman's body, and the physiological changes that occur can alter insulin sensitivity and blood sugar levels. For women with diabetes, maintaining tight blood glucose control is critical to avoid complications for both mother and baby.

Gestational Diabetes

Gestational diabetes (GDM) is a condition that develops during pregnancy, typically in the second or third trimester. It is characterized by high blood sugar levels that occur due to the body's inability to produce enough insulin to meet the increased demands of pregnancy. Women with GDM are at a higher risk of developing Type 2 diabetes later in life, and the condition also increases the risk of pregnancy complications such as **pre-eclampsia**, **macrosomia** (a condition where the baby is born unusually large), and **preterm birth**.

Managing GDM generally involves careful blood glucose monitoring, dietary modifications, and sometimes insulin therapy. If blood sugar levels cannot be controlled with diet and exercise alone, **insulin injections** or **oral medications** (such as **metformin**) may be prescribed.

Insulin Management

For women with pre-existing diabetes (Type 1 or Type 2), **insulin management** during pregnancy is particularly challenging due to the hormonal changes that affect insulin sensitivity. Pregnancy hormones, especially **placental hormones** like **human placental lactogen (hPL)** and **progesterone**, increase insulin resistance in the second and third trimesters.

This means that women with Type 1 diabetes often need to increase their **insulin doses** during pregnancy, and women with Type 2 diabetes may need to start or adjust insulin therapy. It's also important for pregnant women with diabetes to monitor their blood glucose levels more frequently to avoid episodes of **hypoglycemia** (low blood sugar), which can be dangerous for both mother and baby.

Monitoring Blood Glucose Levels

Frequent blood glucose monitoring is crucial for managing diabetes during pregnancy. Women with diabetes should check their blood sugar levels **at least four times a day**—typically fasting, pre-meal, and post-meal. The target blood glucose levels during pregnancy are:

- **Fasting glucose**: 70–95 mg/dL
- **One hour post-meal**: <140 mg/dL
- **Two hours post-meal**: <120 mg/dL

Pregnant women with diabetes also need to monitor their blood pressure regularly, as **hypertension** can complicate pregnancy and increase the risk of **pre-eclampsia**, a dangerous condition characterized by high blood pressure and organ dysfunction.

Diet and Exercise During Pregnancy

Nutrition is particularly important for pregnant women with diabetes. A well-balanced, **diabetic-friendly diet** that includes a variety of healthy foods can help regulate blood sugar levels. Key dietary recommendations include:

- **Small, frequent meals**: Eating smaller meals more often can help prevent large fluctuations in blood sugar levels.
- **Carbohydrate counting**: Understanding how carbohydrates affect blood sugar is essential. Women with diabetes should work with a dietitian to develop a personalized meal plan and learn how to count carbs properly.
- **Healthy fats and proteins**: Incorporating healthy fats (such as omega-3 fatty acids from fish and nuts) and lean proteins can help stabilize blood glucose.
- **Moderate physical activity**: Unless otherwise contraindicated, regular physical activity (such as walking, swimming, or prenatal yoga) can help improve insulin sensitivity and overall health during pregnancy.

Managing Diabetes After Pregnancy

After childbirth, women who had **gestational diabetes** should be monitored for **Type 2 diabetes**, as they are at an increased risk of developing the condition in the years following their pregnancy. For women with pre-existing diabetes, postpartum care involves adjusting insulin therapy and blood sugar management strategies to align with non-pregnant physiology.

Postpartum Blood Sugar Monitoring

Women who had gestational diabetes should have their blood glucose levels checked **within 6–12 weeks** after delivery to determine if they have developed Type 2 diabetes. This is typically done with an **oral glucose tolerance test (OGTT)** or **HbA1c** testing. Ongoing monitoring is essential, as those who have had gestational diabetes have a significantly higher lifetime risk of developing Type 2 diabetes. Women with pre-existing diabetes will likely need to adjust their insulin regimen following childbirth. Hormonal changes during pregnancy often mean that insulin requirements decrease after delivery, so blood sugar monitoring will help adjust insulin doses accordingly. In some cases, women may be able to reduce their insulin doses or even stop insulin therapy after pregnancy.

Breastfeeding and Diabetes

Breastfeeding offers numerous health benefits for both the mother and the baby. For women with diabetes, breastfeeding can help with postpartum weight loss and blood sugar regulation. Studies have shown that **exclusive breastfeeding** can lower the risk of Type 2 diabetes for mothers who had gestational diabetes. However, breastfeeding can also affect blood glucose levels, as it can cause lower blood sugar (hypoglycemia) in some women. Frequent monitoring of blood glucose levels during breastfeeding is important to avoid hypoglycemia and ensure proper nutritional intake for both the mother and the baby.

Risks and Special Considerations for Pregnant Women with Diabetes

Pregnant women with diabetes face several risks, both for themselves and their baby. **Uncontrolled blood sugar** during pregnancy can result in complications such as:

- **Macrosomia** (a larger-than-average baby), which can lead to **difficult delivery, shoulder dystocia,** and an increased likelihood of **cesarean section (C-section).**
- **Preterm labor** and the associated risks for the baby, including **respiratory distress syndrome** and **jaundice.**
- **Congenital malformations**, especially if blood glucose levels are poorly controlled during the first trimester of pregnancy.
- **Pre-eclampsia** (high blood pressure and organ dysfunction), which can cause maternal and fetal complications if left untreated.
- **Neonatal hypoglycemia**, which occurs when the baby's blood sugar drops too low after birth due to high insulin production in response to high maternal blood sugar levels.

Therefore, it's critical that pregnant women with diabetes have close monitoring and a comprehensive care plan to reduce these risks and promote healthy outcomes for both mother and baby.

Conclusion

Managing diabetes during pregnancy requires a careful, comprehensive approach that includes optimizing blood sugar control before pregnancy, vigilant monitoring during pregnancy, and ongoing care after childbirth. With the right medical care, lifestyle modifications, and support from a multidisciplinary healthcare team, most women with diabetes can have a healthy pregnancy and deliver a healthy baby.

However, achieving the best possible outcomes requires attention to detail, a willingness to adapt, and proactive management of the various challenges that diabetes presents throughout the pregnancy journey.

Chapter 27

The Importance of Regular Health Screenings

For individuals living with diabetes, regular health screenings are an essential component of ongoing care. Diabetes can have far-reaching effects on multiple organ systems, making early detection and management of potential complications critical to maintaining health and quality of life. Regular check-ups, eye exams, foot care, kidney function tests, and cardiovascular assessments are all part of a comprehensive strategy to prevent and mitigate the long-term complications associated with diabetes.

In this chapter, we explore the importance of these screenings, how they work, and how proactive management can significantly reduce the risk of complications. Consistent monitoring of diabetes-related health parameters empowers individuals to take charge of their health and avoid potentially devastating outcomes.

Eye Exams: Protecting Vision and Preventing Retinopathy

One of the most significant risks of long-term uncontrolled diabetes is **diabetic retinopathy**, a condition that affects the blood vessels in the eyes and can lead to blindness if left untreated. Retinopathy is often present before any noticeable symptoms appear, making it vital to have regular eye exams to detect the condition early.

What Is Diabetic Retinopathy?

Diabetic retinopathy occurs when high blood glucose levels damage the tiny blood vessels in the retina, the light-sensitive tissue at the back of the eye. Over time, these damaged vessels can leak blood or fluid, causing swelling and affecting vision. In more advanced stages, the body may try to compensate by growing new blood vessels, which are fragile and prone to leakage, leading to even greater visual disturbances.

For individuals with Type 1 diabetes, eye exams should begin within **five years** of diagnosis, and for those with Type 2 diabetes, eye exams should be performed shortly after diagnosis. After the initial exam, most individuals should have a comprehensive eye exam every **1 to 2 years**. However, if retinopathy or other complications are detected, more frequent monitoring may be necessary.

Regular eye exams allow ophthalmologists to identify the early signs of diabetic retinopathy and intervene before the condition progresses. **Laser therapy**, **injections**, or **vitrectomy** (a surgical procedure to remove vitreous gel and blood) can help treat advanced stages of retinopathy and prevent permanent vision loss.

Foot Care: Preventing Diabetic Foot Complications

Diabetes can impair blood circulation and damage the nerves in the feet, increasing the risk of **foot ulcers**, infections, and **amputations**. High blood glucose levels can also contribute to poor healing, making even minor foot injuries more serious.

Diabetic Neuropathy and Its Impact on Foot Health

One of the main contributors to foot problems in people with diabetes is **diabetic neuropathy**, a form of nerve damage that commonly affects the feet. Neuropathy leads to loss of sensation, so a person may not feel pain from cuts, blisters, or other injuries, which increases the risk of infections that can go unnoticed and worsen over time.

Moreover, reduced blood flow (due to peripheral artery disease, or PAD) can make it more difficult for the body to heal infections, leading to longer recovery times and increased risk of severe complications.

Foot Care Recommendations

To prevent foot-related complications, individuals with diabetes should:

- **Inspect their feet daily** for cuts, blisters, redness, or swelling.
- **Wash feet daily** with warm (not hot) water, and thoroughly dry them, especially between the toes, to prevent fungal infections.
- **Moisturize feet** to prevent dry skin and cracks, but avoid moisturizing between the toes, as this can promote fungal growth.
- **Wear well-fitting shoes** and avoid walking barefoot to reduce the risk of injury.
- **Trim toenails carefully** and avoid cutting them too short or rounding the edges, as this can lead to ingrown toenails.

Foot exams should be part of routine diabetes care, typically conducted at every **annual physical** or more frequently if foot issues are present. If nerve damage or poor circulation is detected, further treatments like **medications** for neuropathy or **vascular surgery** to improve circulation may be needed.

Kidney Function: Protecting Against Diabetic Nephropathy

Another common complication of diabetes is **diabetic nephropathy**, a condition that damages the kidneys' filtering system. Over time, high blood sugar levels can damage the blood vessels in the kidneys, impairing their ability to filter waste from the bloodstream. If left untreated, this can lead to **kidney failure**.

Why Kidney Health Is Crucial

The kidneys play a critical role in maintaining overall health by filtering waste, balancing fluid levels, and regulating blood pressure. When diabetic nephropathy progresses, it can lead to **chronic kidney disease (CKD)**, which can eventually require dialysis or a kidney transplant. Early detection of kidney issues is essential because treatments aimed at controlling blood pressure and blood glucose can help slow or even reverse kidney damage.

Screening for Diabetic Nephropathy

The primary tests used to assess kidney function in individuals with diabetes are:

- **Urine albumin-to-creatinine ratio (ACR)**: This test detects excess protein (albumin) in the urine, a sign of kidney damage. Elevated protein levels are one of the earliest indicators of diabetic nephropathy.

- **Serum creatinine and glomerular filtration rate (GFR)**: These tests evaluate how well the kidneys are filtering waste. A decreasing GFR or rising creatinine levels can indicate kidney dysfunction.

People with diabetes should have **annual kidney function tests**, starting shortly after diagnosis, to monitor for early signs of kidney damage. If kidney issues are detected, lifestyle changes (such as **reducing sodium intake** and **increasing hydration**) and medications (such as **angiotensin-converting enzyme (ACE) inhibitors** or **angiotensin receptor blockers (ARBs)**) can help protect the kidneys from further damage.

Cardiovascular Health: Preventing Heart Disease and Stroke

People with diabetes are at a significantly higher risk of **cardiovascular diseases** (CVD), including heart attacks, **stroke**, and

peripheral artery disease. This is due to the combined effects of high blood sugar, high blood pressure, and abnormal cholesterol levels on blood vessel walls.

The Link Between Diabetes and Heart Disease

Chronic high blood sugar levels can damage the blood vessels and increase the buildup of fatty deposits in the arteries, a process called **atherosclerosis**. Over time, this leads to **reduced blood flow**, increasing the likelihood of heart attacks and strokes. Furthermore, many people with diabetes also have other risk factors for CVD, including **hypertension** (high blood pressure) and **dyslipidemia** (high cholesterol).

Cardiovascular Screenings and Tests

To help prevent cardiovascular complications, regular cardiovascular screenings are essential for individuals with diabetes. Key tests include:

- **Blood pressure monitoring**: High blood pressure is a major risk factor for CVD. It is important for people with diabetes to maintain their blood pressure below **140/90 mmHg**.

- **Cholesterol and lipid profile**: Regular testing for total cholesterol, LDL (bad cholesterol), HDL (good cholesterol), and triglycerides is necessary to assess cardiovascular risk.

- **Electrocardiogram (EKG)**: An EKG can help detect any early signs of heart disease, such as arrhythmias (irregular heartbeats) or other electrical abnormalities in the heart.

- **Ankle-brachial index (ABI)**: This test compares blood pressure measurements in the ankle and arm to detect peripheral artery disease, a condition that can result from poor circulation due to diabetes.

Lifestyle modifications, including a **heart-healthy diet**, **regular physical activity**, and **medications** for controlling blood pressure and cholesterol, are essential in managing cardiovascular health. Regular screenings can help identify early signs of heart disease, allowing for timely interventions to reduce the risk of severe cardiovascular events.

The Role of Regular Health Screenings in Preventing Complications

Early detection is key to preventing the progression of diabetes-related complications. Through regular health screenings, individuals with diabetes can identify issues like diabetic retinopathy, neuropathy, nephropathy, and cardiovascular problems before they become severe. With appropriate interventions—whether through **medications**, **lifestyle changes**, or **medical procedures**—complications can often be managed or prevented.

By prioritizing regular check-ups, individuals with diabetes empower themselves to take control of their health and reduce the risk of long-term complications that can significantly impact their quality of life. Early intervention can make all the difference, ensuring that diabetes is managed effectively and that complications are prevented or minimized.

Conclusion

Diabetes requires comprehensive, ongoing care to manage blood sugar levels and prevent complications. Regular health screenings, including eye exams, foot care, kidney function tests, and cardiovascular assessments, play an integral role in the early detection and prevention of complications. By taking a proactive approach to health monitoring, individuals with diabetes can lead longer, healthier lives, minimizing the risk of debilitating conditions and improving their overall well-being. Regular screenings are not just about detecting problems—they are about staying ahead of potential issues, empowering individuals with the knowledge and tools they need to thrive with diabetes.

Chapter 28

Long-Term Complications of Diabetes

Diabetes is often viewed as a condition primarily affecting blood sugar regulation, but its impact extends far beyond this. Over time, uncontrolled or poorly managed diabetes can lead to a range of serious and sometimes debilitating long-term complications. These complications can affect multiple organs and systems in the body, leading to a reduced quality of life and, in extreme cases, disability or death. However, with early detection, appropriate management, and lifestyle changes, it is possible to prevent or delay the onset of these complications.

In this chapter, we will explore some of the most common long-term complications associated with diabetes—**cardiovascular disease, kidney disease, nerve damage**, and **vision problems**—and discuss the strategies that individuals with diabetes can use to reduce their risk and manage these conditions effectively.

Cardiovascular Disease: The Leading Cause of Death in Diabetes

Individuals with diabetes are at a significantly higher risk of developing **cardiovascular disease (CVD)**, which includes conditions such as **heart attacks, stroke**, and **peripheral artery disease (PAD)**. The relationship between diabetes and cardiovascular health is complex and multifactorial, but the underlying mechanism involves the combined effects of high blood glucose, high blood pressure, and elevated cholesterol levels on the blood vessels.

How Diabetes Damages the Heart and Blood Vessels

High blood sugar levels can damage the blood vessels over time, leading to a process known as **atherosclerosis**, where fatty deposits (plaque) build up in the arteries, narrowing and hardening them. This process restricts blood flow and increases the likelihood of **blood clots**, which can block the flow of oxygen-rich blood to the heart or brain, causing a heart attack or stroke. Additionally, individuals with diabetes are more likely to have high blood pressure (hypertension), which further accelerates the damage to blood vessels and increases the risk of heart failure and other cardiovascular problems.

Preventing Cardiovascular Complications

Preventing or delaying cardiovascular complications is one of the most important aspects of managing diabetes. Key strategies include:

- **Controlling blood sugar levels**: Keeping blood glucose within target ranges is essential in preventing the vascular damage that leads to heart disease. Both **HbA1c levels** and **daily blood sugar monitoring** are important tools in managing long-term glucose control.

- **Managing blood pressure**: People with diabetes should aim for a blood pressure of less than **140/90 mmHg**. Lifestyle changes like reducing salt intake, exercising regularly, and losing weight can help lower blood pressure. Medications, such as **ACE inhibitors** and **angiotensin receptor blockers (ARBs)**, may also be prescribed to protect the heart and kidneys.

- **Cholesterol management**: High cholesterol contributes to plaque formation in the arteries. Statins, along with dietary modifications, can help lower LDL cholesterol levels, raising HDL (good) cholesterol and reducing triglycerides.

- **Physical activity**: Regular exercise improves insulin sensitivity, helps control blood sugar levels, and lowers blood pressure and cholesterol, all of which reduce the risk of cardiovascular disease.
- **Quit smoking**: Smoking significantly increases the risk of heart disease and stroke, especially in people with diabetes. Smoking cessation is one of the most beneficial lifestyle changes for improving cardiovascular health.

Kidney Disease: Protecting the Nephrons

Diabetic **nephropathy** (kidney disease) is a common and serious complication of diabetes, affecting the kidneys' ability to filter waste from the blood. Over time, high blood glucose levels can damage the blood vessels in the kidneys, impairing their function and leading to chronic kidney disease (CKD). If left untreated, CKD can progress to **end-stage renal disease (ESRD)**, requiring dialysis or a kidney transplant.

How High Blood Sugar Affects Kidney Function

The kidneys contain millions of tiny blood vessels called **nephrons**, which filter waste and excess fluids from the blood. Chronic high blood sugar levels can cause these blood vessels to become damaged and leaky, allowing protein (such as **albumin**) to pass into the urine. This is one of the first signs of diabetic nephropathy, and if not addressed, it can lead to kidney failure.

The good news is that kidney disease can often be prevented or delayed with early intervention. Effective strategies include:

- **Blood sugar control**: Maintaining normal blood glucose levels reduces the strain on the kidneys and slows the progression of diabetic nephropathy. Both lifestyle changes and medications can help achieve and sustain optimal glucose control.

- **Blood pressure management**: High blood pressure is a major risk factor for kidney disease. Keeping blood pressure within target ranges (generally less than **140/90 mmHg**) is crucial for kidney protection.

- **Reducing protein intake**: In advanced kidney disease, reducing dietary protein can help reduce the kidneys' workload. A dietitian can provide guidance on managing protein consumption.

- **Medications**: **ACE inhibitors** and **ARBs** are commonly prescribed to help protect the kidneys from damage, especially in people with early signs of nephropathy.

- **Regular screening**: People with diabetes should have their **urine albumin-to-creatinine ratio (ACR)** tested annually, as this test can detect early kidney damage. Additionally, regular **creatinine** and **GFR** testing can help track kidney function.

Nerve Damage (Neuropathy): Managing Pain and Preventing Loss of Sensation

Diabetic neuropathy is a type of nerve damage that occurs as a result of prolonged high blood glucose levels. The condition can affect various parts of the body, including the **feet, legs, hands**, and **digestive system**, leading to pain, loss of sensation, and difficulty with motor functions.

How High Blood Sugar Causes Nerve Damage

High blood glucose levels can damage the small blood vessels that supply oxygen and nutrients to the nerves, impairing their function. In addition, high glucose levels may lead to the accumulation of harmful substances that disrupt nerve signaling. The most common form of neuropathy in diabetes is **peripheral neuropathy**, which affects the nerves in the feet and legs. This can lead to numbness, tingling, and, in severe cases, ulcers and infections.

Preventing and Managing Neuropathy

To prevent or manage diabetic neuropathy, several strategies can be employed:

- **Blood sugar control**: Keeping blood glucose levels under control is the best way to prevent nerve damage. The longer blood sugar levels remain elevated, the higher the risk of developing neuropathy.

- **Pain management**: Medications like **antidepressants**, **anticonvulsants**, and **topical treatments** can help manage the pain associated with neuropathy. In some cases, **opioid medications** may be prescribed for severe pain.

- **Foot care**: Since neuropathy often affects the feet, regular foot inspections are essential. People with diabetes should look for cuts, blisters, or infections that may go unnoticed due to loss of sensation.

- **Lifestyle changes**: **Smoking cessation**, **regular exercise**, and a **healthy diet** all contribute to nerve health and can help manage symptoms of neuropathy.

Vision Problems: Protecting Your Eyesight

Diabetes is a leading cause of **vision impairment** and **blindness**. The most common vision problem associated with diabetes is **diabetic retinopathy**, a condition that damages the blood vessels in the retina, the light-sensitive tissue at the back of the eye. Diabetic retinopathy is often asymptomatic in its early stages, making regular eye exams essential for early detection.

How Diabetes Affects Vision

High blood glucose levels can cause the blood vessels in the retina to leak fluid, leading to swelling and vision distortion. Over time, this can result in permanent damage to the retina and vision loss. Additionally, diabetes increases the risk of other eye conditions, such as **glaucoma** and **cataracts**, which can further impair vision.

Preventing Vision Complications

To reduce the risk of diabetic eye problems, individuals with diabetes should:

- **Control blood sugar levels**: Keeping blood glucose levels stable is essential for protecting the blood vessels in the eyes.

- **Regular eye exams**: People with diabetes should have a comprehensive eye exam at least **once a year**, even if they do not experience any symptoms. Early detection of diabetic retinopathy allows for timely interventions to prevent vision loss.

- **Manage blood pressure and cholesterol**: High blood pressure and cholesterol can also affect the blood vessels in the eyes. Managing these risk factors is key to maintaining eye health.

- **Quit smoking**: Smoking increases the risk of eye diseases, including diabetic retinopathy. Quitting smoking can help preserve vision and overall eye health.

Conclusion

Diabetes is a complex disease that can lead to a variety of long-term complications if not properly managed. Cardiovascular disease, kidney disease, nerve damage, and vision problems are among the most common and serious complications associated with diabetes. However, through vigilant blood sugar control, regular health screenings, and lifestyle modifications, individuals with diabetes can significantly reduce their risk of these complications.

Preventing or delaying the onset of long-term complications is not only about managing blood glucose levels but also about adopting a holistic approach to health that includes regular check-ups, a healthy diet, regular exercise, and proper medical care. By taking proactive steps, individuals with diabetes can live longer, healthier lives, minimizing the impact of the disease on their overall well-being.

Chapter 29

Diabetic Retinopathy and Eye Care

Diabetes, a condition primarily affecting blood sugar regulation, has widespread effects on the body, one of which is on the eyes. **Diabetic retinopathy** is one of the most common complications of diabetes and a leading cause of blindness in adults. This condition develops when high blood sugar levels cause damage to the blood vessels in the retina, the part of the eye that detects light and sends visual signals to the brain. Over time, this damage can lead to vision impairment, and without timely intervention, it can result in irreversible blindness.

In this chapter, we will explore the impact of diabetes on eye health, particularly how diabetic retinopathy develops, its stages, and the most effective **prevention** and **early intervention strategies** for preserving vision and managing eye health in people with diabetes.

The Impact of Diabetes on Eye Health

The eye is a delicate organ with a complex system of blood vessels that supply nutrients to its tissues, including the retina. In people with diabetes, high blood sugar levels can cause a series of changes to these blood vessels, leading to a condition known as **diabetic retinopathy**.

How Diabetes Affects the Retina

The retina is made up of light-sensitive cells that play a crucial role in vision. These cells depend on a rich supply of oxygen and nutrients delivered through tiny blood vessels. Over time, high blood sugar can damage the walls of these blood vessels, causing them to leak fluid or blood into the retina. As the disease progresses, new, fragile blood vessels may form in the retina in an attempt to compensate for the damage, but these new vessels are often weak and prone to leaking, which can worsen the problem.

There are two primary mechanisms through which diabetes affects eye health:

- **Hyperglycemia-induced damage**: Elevated blood sugar levels cause changes in the structure of the retinal blood vessels, including thickening of the vessel walls and leakage of fluid. This can lead to swelling in the retina, which impairs its ability to function properly.

- **Oxidative stress**: High blood sugar levels lead to an increase in the production of free radicals, which damage the blood vessels in the retina. This oxidative stress accelerates the development of diabetic retinopathy and other diabetic eye conditions.

The two most common eye conditions linked to diabetes are **diabetic retinopathy** and **diabetic macular edema**. Diabetic macular edema occurs when fluid leaks into the **macula**, the part of the retina responsible for sharp, central vision. This can result in blurry or distorted vision and, if left untreated, may lead to permanent vision loss.

The Stages of Diabetic Retinopathy

Diabetic retinopathy typically develops in stages, with each stage representing the progression of the disease. Early detection and intervention are critical in preventing vision loss. The stages of diabetic retinopathy are:

- **Non-proliferative diabetic retinopathy (NPDR)**: In the early stages, diabetic retinopathy is usually asymptomatic. However, small areas of swelling, bleeding, and hard exudates (fatty deposits) can develop in the retina. This stage is known as NPDR. If blood vessels become weakened and leak fluid into the retina, **macular edema** can occur.

- **Proliferative diabetic retinopathy (PDR)**: In the more advanced stages of diabetic retinopathy, new, abnormal blood vessels begin to form on the retina in an attempt to restore blood flow. However, these new vessels are fragile and can leak blood into the vitreous (the gel-like substance in the eye). This can lead to **retinal detachment**, severe vision impairment, or blindness.

- **Diabetic macular edema (DME)**: Diabetic macular edema is a condition where the macula swells due to the leakage of fluid from damaged blood vessels. It often occurs as a result of NPDR or PDR and can significantly impact central vision, making tasks such as reading and driving difficult. While diabetic retinopathy progresses slowly, it is often asymptomatic in the early stages, which is why **regular eye exams** are crucial for detecting the condition before it leads to vision loss.

Prevention and Early Intervention Strategies for Diabetic Retinopathy

Early intervention is key to preventing or slowing the progression of diabetic retinopathy. The following strategies are essential for reducing the risk of developing diabetic retinopathy and managing the condition effectively.

Blood Sugar Control

The most important factor in preventing diabetic retinopathy is **maintaining good blood sugar control**. Elevated blood sugar levels damage blood vessels over time, and managing glucose levels can prevent or slow the progression of eye damage.

- **Achieving target blood glucose levels**: Keeping blood glucose levels within the recommended target range helps prevent fluctuations that contribute to vascular damage in the retina. Individuals with diabetes should work with their healthcare provider to set realistic blood sugar goals and track their progress using regular blood glucose tests and HbA1c measurements.
- **Continuous monitoring**: For those with Type 1 or Type 2 diabetes, using a **continuous glucose monitor (CGM)** can provide real-time data on glucose levels, allowing for immediate adjustments to diet, exercise, or insulin use.

Blood Pressure and Cholesterol Management

High **blood pressure** and **high cholesterol** are additional risk factors for diabetic retinopathy. Hypertension can accelerate the damage to retinal blood vessels, while high cholesterol can contribute to plaque buildup in the blood vessels, limiting blood flow.

- **Controlling blood pressure**: Keeping blood pressure at or below **140/90 mmHg** is important for preserving eye health. Lifestyle changes such as reducing salt intake, increasing physical activity, and losing weight can help lower blood pressure. Medications may also be prescribed to manage blood pressure.
- **Managing cholesterol levels**: Statin medications may be used to lower cholesterol levels, reducing the risk of atherosclerosis and improving circulation. A heart-healthy diet rich in fiber, healthy fats, and antioxidants can also help maintain healthy cholesterol levels.

Regular Eye Exams

Because diabetic retinopathy often develops without noticeable symptoms, individuals with diabetes should undergo **regular eye exams** to detect early changes in the retina. An annual **dilated eye exam** is recommended for people with Type 1 or Type 2 diabetes, even if they do not experience any vision problems. During these exams, an eye doctor will use specialized equipment to look for signs of retinopathy, including swelling, bleeding, and changes in the blood vessels of the retina.

- **Early detection**: Catching diabetic retinopathy in its early stages (NPDR) is critical, as this is the point at which interventions can be most effective in preventing progression. If any signs of retinopathy are detected, the eye doctor may refer the patient to a retina specialist for further evaluation and treatment.

Managing Diabetic Macular Edema

If diabetic macular edema (DME) develops, early treatment can often preserve vision and prevent further damage to the retina. Treatment options for DME include:

- **Anti-VEGF therapy**: **Anti-vascular endothelial growth factor (anti-VEGF) injections** are commonly used to reduce the growth of abnormal blood vessels and decrease fluid leakage from existing blood vessels in the retina. These injections can significantly improve vision in people with DME.
- **Laser treatment**: **Focal laser photocoagulation** can be used to treat areas of the retina where fluid is leaking. The laser seals the leaky blood vessels, reducing swelling and preventing further vision loss.

- **Corticosteroids**: In some cases, corticosteroid injections or implants may be used to reduce inflammation and fluid leakage in the retina.

Lifestyle Modifications for Eye Health

Maintaining a healthy lifestyle is crucial for preserving eye health and preventing the onset of diabetic retinopathy. The following lifestyle modifications can help reduce the risk of eye complications:

- **Quit smoking**: Smoking accelerates the progression of diabetic retinopathy by damaging blood vessels and increasing the risk of cardiovascular disease. Quitting smoking improves circulation and reduces the risk of vision loss.

- **Regular exercise**: Physical activity helps regulate blood sugar levels, blood pressure, and cholesterol, all of which contribute to eye health. Regular exercise, such as walking, swimming, or cycling, can also improve circulation and reduce the risk of diabetic complications.

- **Healthy diet**: A nutrient-rich diet that includes plenty of **fruits, vegetables, whole grains**, and **lean proteins** can help manage blood glucose levels and reduce the risk of retinopathy. Foods rich in **antioxidants**, such as leafy greens, berries, and nuts, may help protect the retina from oxidative stress.

Managing Comorbidities

Other conditions, such as **kidney disease** and **cardiovascular disease**, can exacerbate diabetic retinopathy. Managing these comorbidities is crucial for overall health and vision preservation. Regular screenings for kidney function and heart health can help identify problems early, allowing for timely interventions.

Conclusion

Diabetic retinopathy is a significant concern for people with diabetes, but with proper management, it is possible to prevent or delay the onset of vision-threatening complications. Maintaining good blood sugar control, managing blood pressure and cholesterol, and undergoing regular eye exams are the cornerstones of eye care in diabetes. Early detection and intervention, including medical treatments such as anti-VEGF therapy and laser surgery, can preserve vision and prevent the progression of diabetic retinopathy.

By adopting a proactive approach to eye health, individuals with diabetes can protect their vision and maintain a higher quality of life, even in the face of this challenging condition.

Chapter 30

Diabetic Neuropathy – Nerve Damage

Diabetic neuropathy is a serious complication of diabetes that occurs when high blood sugar levels cause damage to the nerves throughout the body. The condition most commonly affects the **nerves of the extremities**, such as those in the **feet, legs, hands**, and **arms**, but it can also affect the autonomic nervous system, which controls involuntary body functions like digestion, heart rate, and blood pressure.

Diabetic neuropathy can lead to a wide range of symptoms, from mild tingling or numbness to severe pain, muscle weakness, and organ dysfunction.

In this chapter, we will delve into the causes, symptoms, and management of **diabetic neuropathy**, emphasizing the importance of early detection and intervention. We will also discuss strategies for **prevention**, as well as the crucial role of **foot care** in reducing the risk of serious complications.

Understanding Diabetic Neuropathy

Diabetic neuropathy is a type of nerve damage that occurs as a result of prolonged exposure to high blood sugar levels. Over time, consistently elevated glucose levels can damage the blood vessels that supply oxygen and nutrients to the nerves, particularly in the extremities. This damage impairs the function of the affected nerves, leading to a range of symptoms depending on which type of neuropathy develops.

There are several types of diabetic neuropathy, each affecting different parts of the body:

- **Peripheral neuropathy**: The most common form, affecting the feet, legs, hands, and arms. It typically starts in the toes and works its way up the legs and arms. People with peripheral neuropathy often experience **numbness, tingling, burning sensations**, and **pain**, especially at night.

- **Autonomic neuropathy**: This form of neuropathy affects the autonomic nervous system, which controls involuntary functions such as blood pressure, heart rate, digestion, and bladder control. It can lead to symptoms such as **digestive issues** (nausea, vomiting, diarrhea), **sexual dysfunction, dizziness**, and problems with **temperature regulation**.

- **Proximal neuropathy (diabetic amyotrophy)**: This rare form of neuropathy affects the thighs, hips, and buttocks, causing severe pain, muscle weakness, and difficulty with movement. It can make activities like standing up or walking challenging.

- **Focal neuropathy**: Also known as mononeuropathy, this type of neuropathy affects specific nerves, often causing sudden, sharp pain. It can occur in the **eye, face**, or **pelvis**, and may cause symptoms such as double vision or paralysis of one side of the face.

Causes of Diabetic Neuropathy

The main cause of diabetic neuropathy is **poor blood sugar control** over an extended period. When blood sugar levels remain elevated for long periods, they cause chemical changes in the nerves and blood vessels, leading to nerve damage. Other contributing factors include:

- **High blood pressure**: Elevated blood pressure can damage blood vessels, reducing the blood flow to nerves and exacerbating nerve damage.

- **High cholesterol levels**: Similar to high blood pressure, high cholesterol contributes to poor circulation, which can affect nerve health.
- **Duration of diabetes**: The longer a person has had diabetes, the greater the risk of developing neuropathy. Individuals with Type 1 diabetes may be at risk after 10 or more years, while those with Type 2 diabetes may experience neuropathy sooner.
- **Genetic predisposition**: Some people may have a genetic tendency to develop nerve damage in response to high blood sugar levels.

Other risk factors for diabetic neuropathy include **smoking, obesity**, and **kidney disease**, all of which further complicate blood sugar control and exacerbate nerve damage.

Symptoms of Diabetic Neuropathy

The symptoms of diabetic neuropathy can vary widely, depending on the type of neuropathy and the nerves involved. Common signs and symptoms include:

- **Tingling or "pins and needles" sensation**: Often felt in the feet, legs, hands, or arms, this is one of the early signs of peripheral neuropathy.
- **Numbness**: A feeling of "deadness" or a lack of sensation in the extremities, particularly in the feet and toes. Numbness can increase the risk of injury, as a person may not feel pain from cuts or blisters.
- **Burning or shooting pain**: Many people with peripheral neuropathy experience sharp, shooting pain that can be severe at night. The pain is often described as a burning sensation and can interfere with sleep.
- **Weakness**: Loss of muscle strength can occur, making it difficult to walk, climb stairs, or perform other physical tasks.

- **Loss of balance**: Nerve damage in the feet and legs can impair balance, making it more likely to fall or suffer injuries.
- **Digestive issues**: Autonomic neuropathy can lead to problems such as **nausea**, **vomiting**, **diarrhea**, or **constipation**, caused by nerve damage affecting the digestive tract.
- **Dizziness or fainting**: When autonomic neuropathy affects the nerves that control blood pressure, it can lead to dizziness or fainting, especially when standing up.
- **Sexual dysfunction**: Neuropathy can affect the nerves that control sexual function, leading to erectile dysfunction in men and vaginal dryness or decreased libido in women.

It is important to note that the symptoms of diabetic neuropathy tend to worsen over time, and early intervention is crucial to slowing the progression of the disease.

Prevention of Diabetic Neuropathy

The key to preventing diabetic neuropathy lies in **controlling blood sugar levels** and addressing the risk factors that contribute to nerve damage. The following strategies can significantly reduce the risk of developing diabetic neuropathy:

- **Maintain optimal blood sugar control**: Keeping blood glucose levels within the recommended range is essential for reducing the risk of nerve damage. This involves consistent monitoring of blood sugar levels, following a balanced diet, and taking prescribed medications, including **insulin** or **oral diabetes medications**.
- **Monitor blood pressure and cholesterol**: High blood pressure and high cholesterol can worsen nerve damage, so managing these conditions through medication, diet, and lifestyle changes is vital.

- **Quit smoking**: Smoking reduces circulation and oxygen flow to the nerves, making it more difficult for the body to repair nerve damage. Quitting smoking is one of the most effective ways to prevent further complications.
- **Regular exercise**: Physical activity improves circulation, enhances blood sugar control, and strengthens muscles, all of which help prevent diabetic neuropathy.
- **Healthy diet**: A diet rich in fruits, vegetables, whole grains, lean proteins, and healthy fats can help keep blood sugar levels stable and prevent complications. Additionally, some research suggests that antioxidants, **omega-3 fatty acids**, and **B vitamins** may help protect nerves from damage.

Managing Diabetic Neuropathy

While **prevention** is the best approach, people who already have diabetic neuropathy can take several steps to **manage** their symptoms and slow the progression of nerve damage. Treatment options include:

- **Pain management**: For those suffering from painful neuropathy, medications such as **antidepressants** (amitriptyline, nortriptyline), **anticonvulsants** (gabapentin, pregabalin), or **topical treatments** (capsaicin cream, lidocaine patches) can help relieve nerve pain. In some cases, opioid pain relievers may be prescribed, but these are typically used as a last resort due to their potential for addiction.
- **Physical therapy**: Physical therapy can help improve muscle strength and coordination, reduce pain, and prevent falls. **Occupational therapy** may also be beneficial for those with more advanced neuropathy, helping individuals adapt to daily tasks and maintain independence.

- **Foot care**: One of the most important aspects of managing diabetic neuropathy is **foot care**. Since nerve damage can lead to loss of sensation in the feet, individuals with diabetes may not feel cuts, blisters, or sores, which can become infected. Regular **foot exams** and **proper footwear** are essential to prevent injuries. People with diabetes should also keep their feet clean, dry, and well-moisturized, and avoid walking barefoot.

Foot Care Tips for Diabetic Neuropathy

- Inspect feet daily for cuts, blisters, sores, or signs of infection.
- Wash feet daily with warm water and mild soap, and dry them thoroughly, especially between the toes.
- Avoid hot baths or heating pads, as diminished sensation may make it difficult to sense when the skin is too hot.
- Wear properly fitting shoes and socks to avoid pressure points and blisters. Consider orthotic insoles if necessary.
- Trim toenails carefully, cutting straight across to avoid ingrown nails.
- If you notice any changes in your feet, such as swelling, redness, or ulcers, contact your healthcare provider immediately.
- **Surgical interventions**: In severe cases of diabetic neuropathy, where the damage causes irreversible nerve injury or complications such as foot ulcers or deformities, surgery may be required to correct the issue or manage pain.

Conclusion

Diabetic neuropathy is a common and potentially debilitating complication of diabetes, but it is preventable and manageable with the right approach. Good blood sugar control, regular check-ups, and lifestyle modifications are crucial in preventing nerve damage. Once neuropathy is diagnosed, a combination of medications, physical therapy, and diligent foot care can help manage symptoms and prevent further complications.

By staying vigilant and proactive in managing their diabetes, individuals can reduce the risk of diabetic neuropathy and preserve their quality of life. Regular medical visits, including eye exams, blood tests, and foot checks, are essential components of comprehensive diabetes management, ensuring early detection and effective treatment of any complications that may arise.

Chapter 31

Diabetic Nephropathy – Kidney Health

Diabetic nephropathy is one of the most serious and common complications of diabetes, affecting the kidneys and potentially leading to kidney failure if not properly managed. It occurs when high blood sugar levels damage the blood vessels in the kidneys, impairing their ability to filter waste from the blood. In the long term, this can result in the gradual loss of kidney function, a condition that can progress to **chronic kidney disease** (CKD) and, ultimately, **end-stage renal disease** (ESRD), requiring dialysis or a kidney transplant.

In this chapter, we will explore how **diabetic nephropathy** develops, the **preventive measures** that can be taken to protect kidney health, the **early signs** of kidney damage, and **treatment options** that can slow or reverse the progression of the disease. We will also examine the relationship between **diabetes management** and kidney health, and how individuals with diabetes can reduce their risk of nephropathy through proactive care.

How Diabetes Affects the Kidneys

The kidneys play a vital role in filtering waste products from the blood, regulating fluid balance, and maintaining electrolyte levels. They contain tiny blood vessels called **glomeruli**, which filter out toxins and excess substances from the bloodstream. In healthy kidneys, this filtration process is efficient and selective, ensuring that necessary substances like proteins and blood cells stay in the bloodstream, while waste products and excess fluids are excreted as urine.

In people with **diabetes**, however, prolonged periods of high blood sugar can lead to a series of changes that damage the blood vessels in the kidneys. Here's how the process typically unfolds:

- **High blood sugar**: When blood glucose levels are consistently high, excess glucose is filtered through the kidneys. Over time, the kidneys' filtration system becomes overloaded with glucose, leading to increased pressure on the glomeruli.

- **Damage to blood vessels**: The increased pressure and the toxic effects of glucose cause the walls of the blood vessels to thicken and become scarred. This scarring reduces the kidneys' ability to filter waste effectively.

- **Protein leakage**: As the glomeruli become damaged, they lose their ability to retain proteins like **albumin**, which are normally too large to pass through the filtration system. When protein leaks into the urine, it is referred to as **albuminuria** or **proteinuria**. The presence of protein in the urine is one of the first signs of kidney damage.

- **Progression of kidney damage**: As the kidneys continue to be subjected to high blood sugar levels, they become progressively less efficient at filtering waste. This can lead to the buildup of waste products in the blood, a condition known as **urcmia**. Eventually, kidney function may decline to the point where dialysis or a kidney transplant is necessary.

Preventive Measures for Diabetic Nephropathy

The good news is that **diabetic nephropathy** can be prevented or delayed with proper diabetes management. Keeping blood sugar levels in check, along with addressing other risk factors such as high blood pressure and high cholesterol, is critical in preserving kidney health. Here are some key preventive measures:

- **Maintain blood glucose control**: One of the most effective ways to prevent kidney damage is to manage blood sugar levels effectively. This means adhering to a healthy diet, exercising regularly, and taking prescribed medications (such as insulin or oral diabetes medications) to keep blood glucose levels within the target range. Regular monitoring of blood sugar levels is essential to ensure they are under control and to detect any fluctuations early.

- **Control blood pressure**: High blood pressure (hypertension) is a major risk factor for diabetic nephropathy. Elevated blood pressure places additional strain on the kidneys' blood vessels, speeding up damage. For individuals with diabetes, blood pressure should be kept below 140/90 mmHg, or ideally lower, as recommended by healthcare providers. Common medications used to control blood pressure in people with diabetes include **ACE inhibitors** (such as **lisinopril**) or **angiotensin receptor blockers (ARBs)** (such as **losartan**), which are particularly beneficial for kidney protection.

- **Manage cholesterol levels**: High cholesterol, particularly elevated levels of **LDL cholesterol** (the "bad" cholesterol), can contribute to the narrowing and hardening of the blood vessels, further impairing kidney function. **Statins** are commonly prescribed to people with diabetes to lower cholesterol levels and reduce the risk of cardiovascular complications, including kidney disease.

- **Maintain a healthy weight**: **Obesity** is a significant risk factor for both **diabetes** and **kidney disease**. Maintaining a healthy weight through a balanced diet and regular exercise helps to improve blood sugar control and reduce pressure on the kidneys.

- **Limit alcohol consumption and quit smoking**: Both **alcohol** and **tobacco** have negative effects on kidney function. Smoking, in particular, can narrow the blood vessels and reduce blood flow to the kidneys, accelerating kidney damage. Avoiding smoking and limiting alcohol intake are important lifestyle changes that can help protect kidney health.

- **Stay hydrated**: Adequate hydration is important for kidney function. While it's important to avoid excessive fluid intake, maintaining a balanced level of hydration helps the kidneys filter waste products effectively. Always follow your healthcare provider's recommendations regarding fluid intake.

Early Detection of Diabetic Nephropathy

Detecting diabetic nephropathy early is crucial for preventing the progression of kidney damage. Early signs of kidney damage may not be noticeable, but there are specific tests that can detect nephropathy before symptoms become severe.

- **Urine tests**: One of the most effective ways to detect early kidney damage is through the **urine albumin-to-creatinine ratio (UACR)** test, which measures the amount of **albumin** (a type of protein) in the urine. The presence of albumin in the urine is an early sign of kidney damage. A UACR greater than 30 mg/g indicates the presence of albuminuria, suggesting that the kidneys may be beginning to leak protein. This test is typically performed annually for people with diabetes, starting after five years of diagnosis for Type 1 diabetes and at the time of diagnosis for Type 2 diabetes.

- **Blood tests**: The **serum creatinine test** measures the level of creatinine in the blood, which is a byproduct of muscle metabolism filtered out by the kidneys. Elevated creatinine levels may indicate impaired kidney function. The **estimated glomerular filtration rate (eGFR)**, derived from the serum creatinine test, is used to assess kidney function. An eGFR of 60 mL/min/1.73m^2 or higher is considered normal, while levels below 60 may suggest kidney dysfunction.

- **Blood pressure monitoring**: As high blood pressure is a major risk factor for diabetic nephropathy, regular blood pressure checks are essential. Consistently high blood pressure levels should be managed promptly to prevent kidney damage.

Treatment Options for Diabetic Nephropathy

Once diabetic nephropathy is diagnosed, the goal of treatment is to slow its progression and prevent further kidney damage. While kidney damage from diabetes cannot be reversed, appropriate treatment can help maintain kidney function for as long as possible. The following treatment options are commonly used:

- **Medications to protect the kidneys**: Certain medications can slow the progression of diabetic nephropathy by protecting the kidneys. These include:

  - **ACE inhibitors** or **ARBs**: These drugs are commonly prescribed for people with diabetic nephropathy to help reduce proteinuria (protein in the urine) and protect kidney function. They also help control blood pressure, which is crucial for slowing kidney damage.

  - **SGLT2 inhibitors**: A newer class of diabetes medication, **SGLT2 inhibitors** (such as **empagliflozin** or **canagliflozin**) have shown promise in reducing the risk of kidney disease progression in people with Type 2 diabetes. These medications help control blood sugar levels and may also reduce the risk of kidney failure.

- **Dietary changes**: A kidney-friendly diet is an important aspect of managing diabetic nephropathy. This may involve reducing the intake of **salt**, **potassium**, and **phosphorus**, as well as limiting protein intake to reduce the strain on the kidneys. A **low-protein** diet is often recommended to slow the progression of kidney disease.

- **Dialysis**: In cases of advanced kidney failure, when the kidneys can no longer adequately filter waste products from the blood, **dialysis** may be necessary. Dialysis involves using a machine to remove waste, excess fluids, and salts from the blood. There are two main types of dialysis: **hemodialysis** (where blood is filtered through a machine outside the body) and **peritoneal dialysis** (where the blood is filtered inside the body through a catheter).

- **Kidney transplant**: In severe cases of kidney failure, a **kidney transplant** may be the best option for people with end-stage renal disease. A kidney transplant involves replacing the diseased kidney with a healthy kidney from a donor.

Conclusion

Diabetic nephropathy is a serious complication of diabetes that can lead to kidney failure if not properly managed. Early detection and intervention are key to preventing or delaying the progression of kidney disease. By maintaining **tight blood glucose control**, managing **blood pressure**, addressing **cholesterol levels**, and adopting a **healthy lifestyle**, individuals with diabetes can significantly reduce their risk of developing kidney problems.

Regular monitoring of kidney function through urine tests and blood tests is essential for early detection. If diabetic nephropathy is diagnosed, appropriate treatment options—including medications, dietary changes, and in severe cases, dialysis or a kidney transplant—can help manage the condition and preserve kidney health for as long as possible. With proper care, people with diabetes can live full and healthy lives while managing the risk of nephropathy and other complications.

Chapter 32

Cardiovascular Risk and Diabetes

The link between **diabetes** and **cardiovascular disease** (CVD) is undeniable and represents one of the most critical areas of concern for people living with diabetes. Those with diabetes are at a significantly higher risk of developing heart disease, stroke, and other related complications compared to individuals without diabetes. Understanding the connection between the two, as well as the steps that can be taken to mitigate cardiovascular risk, is essential for effective diabetes management and long-term health.

This chapter explores the mechanisms behind the increased cardiovascular risk in individuals with diabetes and offers practical strategies to reduce that risk, improving both heart and overall health.

Understanding the Connection Between Diabetes and Heart Disease

The relationship between diabetes and cardiovascular disease is complex, and multiple factors contribute to the increased risk of heart-related problems in individuals with diabetes. From **insulin resistance** to **high blood sugar levels**, diabetes affects the cardiovascular system in several critical ways.

Chronic high blood sugar (hyperglycemia) is one of the primary contributors to cardiovascular risk in individuals with diabetes. Over time, poorly controlled blood glucose levels can damage blood vessels and lead to atherosclerosis, which is the buildup of fatty deposits (plaques) in the arteries. This can result in narrowed and hardened arteries, reducing blood flow to vital organs like the heart and brain. The consequences of this can include **heart attacks, stroke**, and other life-threatening conditions.

Insulin resistance, which is a hallmark of Type 2 diabetes, also plays a significant role in increasing cardiovascular risk. When the body becomes resistant to the effects of insulin, the pancreas produces more insulin in an attempt to maintain normal blood sugar levels. Elevated insulin levels can contribute to higher blood pressure, increased levels of harmful fats (such as **triglycerides**), and poor cholesterol profiles—factors that accelerate the development of **atherosclerosis**.

Furthermore, **high blood pressure (hypertension)** is a common co-occurrence in individuals with diabetes. The combination of high blood pressure and diabetes places added strain on the heart and blood vessels, increasing the likelihood of developing **heart disease** or suffering a **stroke**. Uncontrolled blood pressure can further exacerbate the damage caused by high blood glucose, making effective management of both conditions essential.

Another significant factor is the altered **lipid metabolism** in diabetes. Elevated **LDL cholesterol** (often called "bad" cholesterol), high levels of **triglycerides**, and low levels of **HDL cholesterol** (known as "good" cholesterol) contribute to plaque formation in the arteries. The balance of these cholesterol components is often disrupted in people with diabetes, further raising the risk of heart disease.

Additionally, people with diabetes are more likely to have **chronic inflammation**, which is a key contributor to cardiovascular disease. High blood sugar levels increase the production of inflammatory molecules, which can damage blood vessels and promote plaque formation. This inflammatory process accelerates the development of coronary artery disease (CAD) and other heart-related problems.

Steps to Reduce Cardiovascular Risk for People with Diabetes

The good news is that the risks associated with diabetes and cardiovascular disease are largely **preventable** and **manageable** with the right interventions. By focusing on effective blood sugar control, maintaining healthy blood pressure and cholesterol levels, and making heart-healthy lifestyle choices, individuals with diabetes can significantly reduce their cardiovascular risk.

Blood Sugar Control: The Cornerstone of Cardiovascular Health

Effective **blood glucose management** is the foundation of reducing cardiovascular risk in individuals with diabetes. When blood sugar is poorly controlled, it accelerates the process of damage to blood vessels, leading to complications like atherosclerosis. By keeping blood glucose levels within a target range, individuals with diabetes can reduce the long-term risk of heart disease.

Regular blood sugar monitoring is critical. Keeping track of blood glucose through daily self-monitoring and regular HbA1c tests (a marker of long-term blood sugar control) helps ensure that blood glucose stays within an optimal range. For most individuals with diabetes, an HbA1c level of **below 7%** is the target, though this can vary based on individual health circumstances and doctor's recommendations.

In addition to lifestyle modifications, medications play a crucial role in controlling blood sugar levels. Medications such as **insulin** and **oral hypoglycemic agents** (like **metformin, SGLT2 inhibitors**, or **GLP-1 receptor agonists**) help regulate glucose levels. **SGLT2 inhibitors** and

GLP-1 agonists have the added benefit of improving **cardiovascular outcomes**, making them especially valuable for individuals with diabetes at risk for heart disease.

Blood Pressure Control: Managing Hypertension to Protect the Heart

Hypertension (high blood pressure) is a significant risk factor for cardiovascular disease and is common in individuals with diabetes, particularly those with Type 2 diabetes. High blood pressure accelerates the damage to blood vessels, leading to increased risk of heart attack, stroke, and kidney damage.

The **target blood pressure** for most people with diabetes is typically **below 140/90 mmHg**, though individual goals may vary. Achieving this target requires a combination of lifestyle modifications and, in some cases, medication.

Lifestyle changes play a significant role in controlling blood pressure. Regular **physical activity** can help lower blood pressure, as can reducing **salt intake** and adopting a **heart-healthy diet**, such as the **DASH diet** (Dietary Approaches to Stop Hypertension), which emphasizes fruits, vegetables, whole grains, lean proteins, and low-fat dairy products.

In some cases, medications such as **ACE inhibitors, ARBs** (angiotensin receptor blockers), **beta-blockers**, or **calcium channel blockers** may be prescribed to help control blood pressure and protect the heart. **ACE inhibitors** and **ARBs** are particularly beneficial because they also protect the kidneys, another vital organ often affected by diabetes.

Cholesterol Management: Balancing Lipid Levels

Elevated **cholesterol levels** are another major contributor to cardiovascular risk in people with diabetes. Uncontrolled diabetes leads to an imbalance in lipid metabolism, with increased **LDL cholesterol** (bad cholesterol) and **triglycerides**, and decreased **HDL cholesterol** (good cholesterol).

Managing **lipid levels** is critical for reducing the risk of heart disease. A healthy, **heart-healthy diet** rich in **omega-3 fatty acids** (from fishlike salmon), **fiber** (from whole grains, fruits, and vegetables), and **monounsaturated fats** (like olive oil and avocados) can help lower LDL cholesterol and triglyceride levels while boosting HDL cholesterol. In addition to dietary changes, **statins** are commonly prescribed to lower LDL cholesterol and reduce the risk of cardiovascular events. Medications like **ezetimibe** and **PCSK9 inhibitors** can also help lower cholesterol levels when statins are not enough.

Exercise: A Powerful Tool for Heart Health

Physical activity is one of the most effective ways to manage diabetes and reduce cardiovascular risk. Regular exercise helps improve **insulin sensitivity**, lower **blood sugar levels**, reduce **blood pressure**, and improve **cholesterol levels**. It also helps with **weight management**, which is a key component of overall cardiovascular health.

Both **aerobic exercise** (such as walking, cycling, swimming, or jogging) and **strength training** (using weights or resistance bands) are beneficial for heart health. Aim for at least **150 minutes of moderate-intensity aerobic activity per week** or **75 minutes of vigorous-intensity**

aerobic activity. Incorporating strength training exercises at least twice a week is also beneficial for improving metabolism and muscle health.

Exercise also helps combat the effects of **obesity**, which is a common risk factor for cardiovascular disease in people with diabetes. Even **modest weight loss** (5–10% of total body weight) can improve blood pressure, cholesterol, and blood sugar levels, significantly reducing the risk of heart disease.

Weight Management: Reducing Excess Weight to Protect the Heart

Maintaining a **healthy weight** is crucial for reducing cardiovascular risk in individuals with diabetes. Obesity, particularly **visceral fat** (fat around the abdomen), is strongly associated with insulin resistance, high blood pressure, high cholesterol, and increased risk of heart disease. Adopting a balanced, calorie-controlled diet rich in **whole foods** and engaging in regular physical activity can help promote **weight loss** and improve overall health. Even a small amount of weight loss can have a profound impact on cardiovascular risk, improving **insulin sensitivity**, lowering **blood pressure**, and improving **lipid profiles**.

Lifestyle Modifications: A Holistic Approach to Heart Health

In addition to managing blood sugar, blood pressure, cholesterol, and weight, there are several **lifestyle modifications** that can help reduce cardiovascular risk:

- **Quit smoking**: Smoking is one of the most significant risk factors for heart disease and stroke. It accelerates the process of **atherosclerosis** and increases the risk of blood clotting, further complicating the cardiovascular risk for individuals with diabetes. Quitting smoking is one of the most impactful actions anyone can take to protect their heart.

- **Limit alcohol consumption**: Excessive alcohol intake can raise **blood pressure**, contribute to **weight gain**, and worsen **blood sugar control**. Limiting alcohol intake to **moderate levels** (one drink per day for women and two for men) is recommended to protect heart health.
- **Manage stress**: Chronic stress can negatively affect blood pressure and overall heart health. Practices like **mindfulness meditation**, **yoga**, and **deep breathing exercises** can help manage stress and improve emotional well-being.

In conclusion, the connection between **diabetes** and **cardiovascular disease** is strong, but with the right **management strategies**, individuals with diabetes

Chapter 33

Technological Advances in Diabetes Care

The rapid evolution of **technology** has dramatically transformed the way we manage diabetes. From **wearable devices** to **artificial pancreas systems**, cutting-edge innovations are not only improving the day-to-day management of the disease but also holding the potential to revolutionize treatment approaches in the near future. As diabetes care continues to progress, technological tools will play an increasingly critical role in helping individuals manage their blood sugar levels, track their health data, and even reduce the burden of the disease.

This chapter explores the impact of **technology** on diabetes care, focusing on the role of **wearables**, **artificial pancreas systems**, **apps**, and the promising future trends in **diabetes monitoring** and **treatment**.

The Role of Wearables in Diabetes Management

One of the most exciting technological advancements in diabetes care has been the development of **wearable devices**. These devices, which include **continuous glucose monitors (CGMs)**, **smartwatches**, and **fitness trackers**, have revolutionized the way individuals with diabetes manage their condition.

Continuous Glucose Monitors (CGMs) are among the most significant technological breakthroughs in diabetes care. Unlike traditional methods of monitoring blood sugar, which require fingersticks multiple times a day, CGMs provide real-time, continuous glucose readings throughout the day and night. By using a small sensor inserted under the skin, a CGM measures glucose levels in the interstitial fluid, sending data to a mobile device or receiver. This allows individuals with diabetes to track their blood glucose levels constantly, providing immediate feedback and helping to identify trends that may require intervention.

The **advantages of CGMs** are numerous. First, they provide **real-time data**, allowing individuals to make timely adjustments to their diet, exercise, or medication. Second, CGMs can alert the wearer to dangerous **blood sugar fluctuations**, including both **hypoglycemia (low blood sugar)** and **hyperglycemia (high blood sugar)**, enabling early intervention before a crisis occurs. CGMs can also improve overall **glucose control**, as users have a clearer picture of their blood sugar levels throughout the day and can better manage fluctuations.

In addition to glucose monitors, **wearable fitness trackers** such as **Fitbit** and **Apple Watch** play a vital role in diabetes management. These devices monitor daily physical activity, heart rate, sleep patterns, and even stress levels.

For individuals with diabetes, staying active and managing stress are essential components of maintaining healthy blood sugar levels. Wearable devices can track how exercise impacts blood sugar, provide motivation for physical activity, and help monitor overall health metrics. Moreover, many modern wearables now have **integration features** that connect with **diabetes management apps** and other medical devices, creating a comprehensive and user-friendly ecosystem for managing the condition.

Artificial Pancreas Systems: The Next Step in Diabetes Management

One of the most groundbreaking advances in diabetes technology is the development of the **artificial pancreas system** (APS). The artificial pancreas is designed to **automatically regulate blood glucose levels**, combining the functions of an insulin pump and continuous glucose monitoring in a closed-loop system. This system, also known as **closed-loop insulin delivery**, mimics the function of a healthy pancreas by continuously monitoring blood sugar and automatically delivering insulin or glucagon as needed to maintain glucose levels within a safe range. The key components of an artificial pancreas system include:

- **Continuous Glucose Monitor (CGM)**: A CGM tracks blood glucose levels in real-time.

- **Insulin Pump**: An insulin pump delivers a continuous flow of insulin to the body throughout the day.

- **Algorithms and Software**: Advanced algorithms process the data from the CGM and determine the appropriate insulin dose, automatically adjusting the insulin delivery from the pump.

Benefits of artificial pancreas systems include better overall **blood glucose control**, fewer episodes of **hypoglycemia**, and the ability to reduce the burden of daily diabetes management. This system is particularly beneficial for individuals with **Type 1 diabetes**, who need to monitor their glucose levels closely and frequently adjust their insulin doses.

Currently, the FDA has approved several hybrid artificial pancreas systems, which automatically adjust basal insulin levels, while the user is still required to give **bolus doses** at mealtime. However, the goal is to develop fully automated systems that do not require any user input, allowing the **artificial pancreas** to function just like a healthy human pancreas, with minimal intervention from the user.

Diabetes Management Apps: Empowering People to Take Control

With the increasing prevalence of **smartphones** and **mobile applications**, **diabetes management apps** have become an essential tool in the daily lives of people with diabetes. These apps help users track their blood glucose levels, diet, exercise, medication, and other important health metrics, empowering individuals to take control of their condition. Many diabetes management apps are designed to **sync with wearables** like CGMs, insulin pumps, and fitness trackers, providing a centralized platform where all health data can be monitored in real-time.

For example, apps like **MySugr** and **Carb Manager** allow users to log their food intake, track their insulin usage, and monitor their exercise routines. These apps also provide helpful insights, such as recommending adjustments to meal plans based on blood sugar trends or offering educational tips on managing the condition.

Data analytics and **personalized recommendations** are becoming increasingly important features of diabetes apps. Some apps can analyze a user's historical data and provide tailored advice on improving blood sugar control, such as suggesting changes in insulin dosing or recommending meal plans to avoid blood sugar spikes. This level of customization and real-time feedback has the potential to improve **glycemic control** and reduce complications associated with poorly managed diabetes.

Moreover, many diabetes apps offer **integration with telemedicine platforms**, enabling users to share their data directly with healthcare providers. This allows for more efficient and proactive care, as healthcare providers can monitor their patients' progress remotely, provide timely interventions, and adjust treatment plans when necessary.

Future Trends in Diabetes Monitoring and Treatment

As technology continues to advance, the future of diabetes care looks increasingly promising. In addition to the developments in wearables, artificial pancreas systems, and diabetes management apps, several key trends are shaping the future of diabetes monitoring and treatment.

Non-Invasive Blood Glucose Monitoring

One of the most highly anticipated innovations in diabetes care is the development of **non-invasive blood glucose monitoring**. Current CGMs require a small sensor to be inserted under the skin, but researchers are working on technologies that can measure glucose levels through other means, such as **infrared spectroscopy**, **optical sensors**, or even **breath analysis**. If successful, non-invasive monitoring would eliminate the need for invasive sensors, making blood glucose testing easier, more comfortable, and accessible.

Personalized Medicine and AI

With the rise of **artificial intelligence (AI)** and **machine learning**, personalized medicine is becoming a reality for individuals with diabetes. AI algorithms can analyze vast amounts of data from multiple sources, including blood glucose readings, genetic information, lifestyle factors, and even environmental influences, to create highly personalized treatment plans. For example, AI could help optimize **insulin dosing**, predict blood sugar fluctuations, or suggest dietary changes based on individual patterns.

Additionally, **genetic testing** may allow for more precise targeting of diabetes treatments, enabling healthcare providers to tailor therapies to the genetic makeup of the individual. This approach could significantly improve treatment outcomes and reduce the risk of complications.

Improved Insulin Delivery Systems

Insulin delivery systems are also undergoing significant advancements. In addition to the artificial pancreas systems mentioned earlier, **smart insulin pens** are becoming more common. These pens can record insulin doses, calculate bolus amounts based on blood glucose readings, and even send data to an app for tracking purposes. Furthermore, researchers are exploring the development of **biologic insulin** and **insulin patches**, which could provide more convenient and effective ways of delivering insulin.

Gene Therapy and Regenerative Medicine

In the long term, **gene therapy** and **regenerative medicine** may offer potential cures for diabetes. Advances in stem cell therapy and gene editing technologies like **CRISPR** are being explored as possible treatments for both Type 1 and Type 2 diabetes. The goal is to repair or replace damaged insulin-producing beta cells in the pancreas, potentially offering a permanent solution to the disease. Although these technologies are still in their early stages, they represent an exciting frontier in diabetes care.

Conclusion

The role of **technology** in diabetes care is expanding rapidly, and innovations such as wearables, artificial pancreas systems, and diabetes management apps are already improving the lives of millions of people with diabetes. These advances offer greater convenience, better glucose control, and the potential for more personalized treatment options. As we look toward the future, emerging trends in non-invasive monitoring, AI-driven personalized medicine, and regenerative therapies may bring us closer to a world where diabetes is more easily managed and even cured.

By embracing these technological advancements, individuals with diabetes will have more tools at their disposal to take control of their condition and improve their health outcomes. The future of diabetes care is not just about managing the disease—it's about **thriving** with it, and technology will continue to be a vital partner in that journey.

Chapter 34

Stem Cell Research and Potential Cures

The search for a **cure for diabetes** has been a long-standing pursuit in the medical community, particularly for **Type 1 diabetes**, where the immune system attacks and destroys the insulin-producing beta cells in the pancreas. For decades, the focus has been on better management strategies, medications, and lifestyle modifications. However, in recent years, the potential of **stem cell research** to regenerate beta cells and restore normal insulin production has opened up new possibilities for a **cure**. This chapter delves into the exciting field of stem cell research and its potential to provide a permanent solution for both **Type 1** and **Type 2 diabetes**.

What Are Stem Cells?

Stem cells are unique cells that have the remarkable ability to develop into many different types of cells in the body. They are often referred to as **undifferentiated cells**, meaning they can transform into specialized cell types, such as muscle cells, nerve cells, or even insulin-producing beta cells. Stem cells are primarily classified into two main categories:

- **Embryonic stem cells (ESCs)**: These stem cells come from embryos and have the potential to become any type of cell in the body. However, their use in research raises ethical concerns.

- **Adult stem cells (ASCs)**: These stem cells are found in various tissues in the body, such as bone marrow or adipose (fat) tissue, and are typically more limited in what types of cells they can transform into. **Induced pluripotent stem cells (iPSCs)**, a form of adult stem cells, are engineered in the lab to become pluripotent, similar to embryonic stem cells, without the ethical issues associated with using embryos.

Stem cells hold enormous promise in the treatment of many diseases because of their ability to regenerate tissues that are damaged or destroyed. In the case of **Type 1 diabetes**, the goal is to **replenish** the damaged **beta cells** in the pancreas, which would potentially cure the disease by restoring the body's natural ability to produce insulin.

Stem Cell Therapy for Type 1 Diabetes

The central challenge in **Type 1 diabetes** is that the body's immune system mistakenly attacks and destroys its insulin-producing **beta cells** in the pancreas. The result is that people with Type 1 diabetes are unable to produce insulin naturally, which leads to high blood sugar levels and the need for external insulin injections.

Stem cell-based therapy offers a potential solution by creating new insulin-producing cells, essentially **replacing** the beta cells that were destroyed. The concept is simple in theory: scientists aim to derive functional beta cells from stem cells and transplant them into a patient's pancreas, thereby restoring insulin production and **normalizing blood glucose levels**.

Recent breakthroughs have demonstrated that stem cells can be coaxed into becoming **beta-like cells** in the laboratory. These cells can secrete insulin in response to glucose levels, which is a key feature of the natural beta cells found in a healthy pancreas. However, turning these cells into fully functional, long-lasting beta cells that will not be rejected by the body and that can function in harmony with the immune system remains a significant challenge.

Scientists have made tremendous strides in recent years toward developing stem cell therapies that may eventually lead to a cure for Type 1 diabetes. Key developments include:

- **Generation of Beta Cells from Stem Cells**: Researchers have successfully generated insulin-producing beta-like cells from **human pluripotent stem cells (hPSCs)**, which can be derived from both **embryonic stem cells (ESCs)** and **induced pluripotent stem cells (iPSCs)**. These beta-like cells can secrete insulin when exposed to glucose, just as natural beta cells would. However, the challenge remains in creating these cells on a large scale and ensuring that they work reliably over time.

- **Immune Protection for Transplanted Cells**: One of the most significant hurdles in using stem cells for diabetes therapy is ensuring that the newly generated beta cells are not attacked by the immune system. Since Type 1 diabetes is an **autoimmune disease**, where the body's immune system attacks and destroys beta cells, researchers are exploring ways to **protect** these stem cells after transplantation. One promising approach is to encapsulate the cells in a **protective layer** that prevents immune system cells from attacking them, allowing the newly formed beta cells to survive and function.

- **In vivo Reprogramming**: Instead of generating beta cells in the laboratory and transplanting them, another potential approach involves using stem cells to **reprogram existing cells** in the body into functional beta cells. For example, researchers have been exploring ways to **convert liver cells** into insulin-producing beta-like cells. This approach could avoid the need for **stem cell transplants** and reduce the risk of immune rejection.

- **Gene Editing Technologies (CRISPR)**: Another cutting-edge technology that holds great potential for stem cell therapy in diabetes is **gene editing**. Using techniques such as **CRISPR-Cas9**, researchers can alter the DNA of stem cells to enhance their ability to become insulin-producing beta cells or to make them more resistant to immune attack. By making precise genetic modifications, scientists hope to improve the effectiveness and safety of stem cell-based therapies for diabetes.

Challenges in Stem Cell Therapy for Diabetes

While the potential of stem cell-based therapies for Type 1 diabetes is promising, significant challenges remain:

- **Scalability**: Creating large quantities of functional beta cells from stem cells is a difficult and costly process. Scaling up these methods to produce enough cells for transplantation in humans is a critical step in advancing stem cell-based therapies.

- **Immune Rejection**: Even if stem cells can be derived from the patient's own tissue (as in the case of **iPSCs**), the risk of **immune rejection** remains a concern. Since diabetes is an autoimmune condition, the immune system may attack the newly generated beta cells. Researchers are working on techniques to **immune-protect** these transplanted cells, such as using **encapsulation** technologies or genetically modifying the stem cells to be less detectable by the immune system.

- **Long-Term Functionality**: A major challenge in stem cell research is ensuring that the beta cells derived from stem cells are not only capable of producing insulin in response to blood sugar levels but also that they can do so for a long period of time without losing their functionality.

Ensuring the longevity and **durability** of stem cell-derived beta cells is essential for developing a viable cure for Type 1 diabetes.

- **Ethical Concerns**: The use of **embryonic stem cells** raises ethical concerns, as obtaining these cells involves the destruction of human embryos. While **iPSCs** have alleviated some of these concerns by offering an alternative source of pluripotent stem cells, the ethical debate surrounding stem cell research remains a topic of ongoing discussion.

How Close Are We to a Cure?

While **stem cell therapy** offers enormous promise for the future, we are still a long way from a universally available cure for **Type 1 diabetes**. Clinical trials are ongoing, and researchers continue to make significant progress in understanding how stem cells can be used to generate insulin-producing cells. However, several key challenges must be overcome before stem cell-based therapies can be widely used as a practical treatment option.

Some recent clinical trials have shown encouraging results, with patients receiving transplants of stem cell-derived beta cells experiencing improved blood sugar control. But these therapies are still in the **experimental stages**, and further research is needed to determine their long-term effectiveness and safety. Moreover, the **cost** of stem cell therapies and the availability of donor cells remain practical barriers that need to be addressed.

Future Outlook: A Multi-Pronged Approach

Despite the challenges, the future of stem cell therapy for diabetes is promising. With continued advancements in **genetic engineering, immune protection strategies**, and **cell manufacturing**, researchers believe that stem cell-based therapies may eventually provide a cure for Type 1 diabetes. However, this will likely be part of a broader, **multi-pronged approach** that combines stem cell therapy with **personalized medicine**, **immune-modulation treatments**, and **lifestyle interventions**. While a definitive cure for Type 1 diabetes remains a goal for the future, the exciting progress being made in **stem cell research** holds great promise for improving the lives of millions of people with diabetes.

In the meantime, ongoing research continues to enhance our understanding of the disease and its management, bringing us closer to a world where diabetes is no longer a lifelong condition but a manageable and treatable illness.

Conclusion

Stem cell research is at the forefront of innovative strategies to cure Type 1 diabetes, and though we are still in the early stages of clinical application, the progress made so far is promising. Through a combination of **genetic engineering**, **immune protection**, and **reprogramming existing cells**, scientists are steadily moving toward the goal of providing a functional cure for diabetes. The journey from laboratory research to clinical application may take time, but the potential benefits of stem cell therapy—ranging from **long-term insulin production** to the restoration of normal glucose metabolism—offer hope for a future without diabetes.

As research continues to unfold, patients, researchers, and healthcare professionals will likely see a convergence of new technologies and treatment modalities, pushing us closer to a **cure** for Type 1 diabetes and improving the overall quality of life for those living with the disease.

Chapter 35

The Role of the Gut Microbiome in Diabetes

In recent years, a growing body of research has highlighted the profound influence of the **gut microbiome** on human health, including its impact on **insulin sensitivity** and the development of **diabetes**. The gut microbiome refers to the complex community of trillions of microorganisms—bacteria, viruses, fungi, and other microbes—that reside in the gastrointestinal tract. These microorganisms play a crucial role in digestion, immune function, and the regulation of metabolic processes. The relationship between the gut microbiome and **diabetes** is an area of intense research, offering potential new strategies for managing and even preventing the disease.

In this chapter, we will explore how the **gut microbiome** influences **insulin sensitivity**, the development of both **Type 1 and Type 2 diabetes**, and how future research into probiotics and diet may provide novel tools for diabetes management.

The Gut Microbiome and Insulin Sensitivity

The gut microbiome plays a pivotal role in regulating various metabolic processes, including those involved in **insulin sensitivity**. Insulin sensitivity refers to how effectively the body responds to insulin, the hormone responsible for helping cells absorb glucose from the bloodstream. In individuals with **insulin resistance**, a condition commonly associated with **Type 2 diabetes**, the body's cells become less responsive to insulin, leading to higher blood glucose levels.

Research has shown that **imbalances in the gut microbiome**—also known as **dysbiosis**—can contribute to the development of **insulin resistance** and metabolic dysfunction. The gut microbiome influences **insulin sensitivity** through several mechanisms:

- **Inflammation**: An imbalanced gut microbiome can promote **chronic low-grade inflammation**. Certain gut bacteria produce substances known as **lipopolysaccharides (LPS)**, which can trigger inflammatory pathways in the body. This inflammation can interfere with the action of insulin, leading to **insulin resistance** and impaired glucose metabolism.

- **Short-Chain Fatty Acids (SCFAs)**: Beneficial gut bacteria ferment dietary fiber into **short-chain fatty acids (SCFAs)**, such as acetate, propionate, and butyrate. SCFAs are critical for regulating **insulin sensitivity**, as they help maintain a healthy balance of gut hormones that influence glucose metabolism. SCFAs also have anti-inflammatory properties, reducing the systemic inflammation associated with insulin resistance.

- **Gut-Brain Axis**: The gut microbiome communicates with the **central nervous system** through the **gut-brain axis**, a bidirectional communication system that links the gastrointestinal tract with the brain. This communication affects **appetite regulation**, **energy balance**, and **glucose metabolism**, all of which are influenced by insulin sensitivity. Dysbiosis can disrupt this communication, leading to impaired metabolic control.

- **Metabolism of Bile Acids**: Gut microbes also play a role in the metabolism of **bile acids**, which are involved in regulating glucose and lipid metabolism. Disruptions in bile acid metabolism caused by an unhealthy microbiome can exacerbate insulin resistance and increase the risk of metabolic diseases like diabetes.

These findings underscore the importance of a healthy and balanced gut microbiome in maintaining **insulin sensitivity** and preventing the onset of **Type 2 diabetes**. The intricate relationship between gut health and metabolic function suggests that **gut-targeted therapies** could become an integral part of managing and potentially reversing diabetes.

Gut Microbiome and Type 2 Diabetes

Type 2 diabetes is characterized by **insulin resistance**, a condition in which the body's cells become less responsive to insulin. This resistance results in elevated blood glucose levels and a cascade of metabolic disturbances. The role of the **gut microbiome** in the development of Type 2 diabetes is a rapidly expanding area of research. Studies have shown that individuals with Type 2 diabetes often have a distinct microbiome compared to healthy individuals. Key differences include:

- **Decreased microbial diversity**: People with Type 2 diabetes often have a less diverse gut microbiome, which is thought to contribute to insulin resistance and metabolic dysfunction. A diverse microbiome is important for maintaining gut health and metabolic homeostasis.

- **Altered microbial composition**: Certain bacteria, such as those from the **Firmicutes** and **Bacteroidetes** phyla, are found in higher or lower abundance in individuals with Type 2 diabetes. Some bacteria produce metabolites like **SCFAs**, which are linked to improved insulin sensitivity, while others may produce **inflammatory molecules** that exacerbate insulin resistance.

- **Gut permeability (Leaky Gut)**: Dysbiosis can also affect the integrity of the **gut lining**, leading to increased **intestinal permeability** or **leaky gut**. This allows harmful substances, such as **endotoxins** from gut bacteria, to enter the bloodstream, triggering inflammation and further impairing insulin signaling.

While the exact mechanisms linking the microbiome to Type 2 diabetes are still being studied, evidence suggests that **gut health** is a key factor in the development and progression of the disease.

Gut Microbiome and Type 1 Diabetes

While much of the research on the gut microbiome has focused on **Type 2 diabetes**, there is also emerging evidence that the microbiome may play a role in the development of **Type 1 diabetes**. Type 1 diabetes is an autoimmune disease in which the body's immune system attacks and destroys the insulin-producing beta cells in the pancreas. Some studies suggest that:

- **Gut microbiome imbalances** may influence immune system function and contribute to the onset of autoimmune diseases, including Type 1 diabetes. For example, certain gut bacteria may trigger immune responses that lead to the destruction of beta cells in genetically predisposed individuals.

- **Early-life microbiome development**: The development of the gut microbiome in early childhood may influence the risk of autoimmune diseases later in life. Studies have shown that an **unbalanced microbiome** in infancy, possibly due to factors like **antibiotic use, caesarean section birth**, or **lack of breastfeeding**, may increase the risk of developing Type 1 diabetes.

- **Immune modulation by the microbiome**: The gut microbiome can influence the balance of immune cells in the body. Dysbiosis may lead to an overactive immune response, which could increase the risk of autoimmune diseases like Type 1 diabetes.

Although the relationship between the gut microbiome and Type 1 diabetes is still being explored, this area of research holds promise for identifying potential **preventive measures** or **therapeutic interventions**.

Probiotics and Gut Health in Diabetes Management

Given the significant role of the gut microbiome in insulin sensitivity and glucose metabolism, **probiotics**—live beneficial microorganisms—have emerged as a potential therapeutic option for managing diabetes. Probiotics may help **restore gut microbiome balance** and improve **insulin sensitivity**, potentially reducing the risk of Type 2 diabetes and improving management of the disease.

Probiotics can:

- **Increase SCFA production**: As mentioned earlier, SCFAs are essential for maintaining insulin sensitivity. Probiotics may promote the growth of beneficial bacteria that produce these compounds, helping to regulate glucose metabolism and reduce inflammation.

- **Reduce systemic inflammation**: Probiotics can help balance the immune response in the gut, potentially reducing **low-grade inflammation** that contributes to insulin resistance.

- **Enhance gut barrier function**: Probiotics may improve the integrity of the **gut lining**, reducing gut permeability and preventing the entry of harmful substances into the bloodstream.

Several studies have investigated the use of probiotics in managing diabetes, with some promising results. For instance, some clinical trials have shown that specific strains of probiotics can improve **blood sugar control** and **insulin resistance** in people with Type 2 diabetes.

Diet and the Microbiome in Diabetes Management

Diet plays a crucial role in shaping the gut microbiome, and certain dietary patterns can support **gut health** and **insulin sensitivity**. The adoption of a **high-fiber diet** rich in fruits, vegetables, legumes, and whole grains can promote the growth of beneficial gut bacteria and increase the production of SCFAs.

Additionally, **prebiotics**—non-digestible food components that stimulate the growth of beneficial microbes—can help nourish the microbiome and further enhance its beneficial effects on glucose metabolism. Foods high in prebiotics include **garlic**, **onions**, **bananas**, and **asparagus**.

The **Mediterranean diet**, which emphasizes plant-based foods, healthy fats, and moderate consumption of lean proteins, has been associated with improved metabolic health and a more diverse gut microbiome. **Fermented foods**, such as yogurt, kefir, kimchi, and sauerkraut, are also rich in probiotics and can support gut health. Future research is likely to focus on identifying specific **dietary interventions** that can help modify the gut microbiome to improve **insulin sensitivity** and prevent or manage diabetes. Personalized nutrition, taking into account individual microbiome profiles, may become a key strategy in **diabetes management**.

Future Research and Clinical Applications

While the connection between the gut microbiome and diabetes is becoming clearer, much more research is needed to fully understand the mechanisms at play. Future studies will likely explore:

- The development of **microbiome-based therapies**, such as **probiotic supplements** or **fecal microbiota transplants**, to improve **insulin sensitivity** and treat or prevent diabetes.

- The role of the **gut-brain axis** in regulating metabolic health, and how interventions that target this pathway could help manage **Type 1** and **Type 2 diabetes**.

- The use of **genetic analysis** to better understand the **gut microbiome** and its interactions with human genetics, enabling **personalized treatment** approaches based on an individual's microbiome composition.

As research advances, it is likely that **microbiome-based interventions** will become a vital part of **diabetes prevention and management**, providing patients with new tools to manage their condition more effectively.

Conclusion

The emerging field of **gut microbiome research** has the potential to transform how we understand and manage **diabetes**. With growing evidence that the gut microbiome plays a central role in **insulin sensitivity**, glucose metabolism, and inflammation, it offers a new frontier for diabetes treatment. **Probiotics, dietary interventions**, and potentially even **fecal microbiota transplants** may soon play a key role in managing diabetes, offering new avenues for therapy that focus on **gut health** and **microbial balance**.

As we continue to uncover the intricate connections between the gut microbiome and metabolic health, we may see the development of more personalized, effective strategies for preventing, managing, and even reversing **Type 2 diabetes**. With continued research, the role of the **gut microbiome** in diabetes management may become an integral part of our approach to tackling this global health challenge.

Chapter 36

Advances in Diabetes Vaccines

In the field of **diabetes research**, one of the most exciting areas of development is the potential for **vaccines** to prevent or treat the disease. While vaccines are primarily known for their role in preventing infectious diseases, recent scientific advancements have led to the exploration of vaccines aimed at **modulating the immune system** in ways that could prevent or reverse the course of **Type 1 diabetes** and even help in the management of **Type 2 diabetes**. This chapter will delve into the latest research on **diabetes vaccines**, the science behind **immune modulation**, and how these vaccines could potentially change the way we approach diabetes treatment in the future.

The Need for Diabetes Vaccines

Diabetes, particularly **Type 1 diabetes**, is an autoimmune condition where the body's immune system mistakenly attacks its own insulin-producing cells in the **pancreas**, known as **beta cells**. As of now, there is no cure for Type 1 diabetes, and treatment revolves around lifelong insulin therapy. Similarly, while **Type 2 diabetes** is primarily linked to **insulin resistance** and lifestyle factors, researchers are exploring vaccines to prevent its progression or help reverse insulin resistance in at-risk populations.

The **rising prevalence** of diabetes worldwide, along with its impact on public health, makes the development of vaccines a promising and urgent goal. By targeting the **immune system**, vaccines could potentially stop the autoimmune attack that destroys beta cells in Type 1 diabetes or improve the body's response to insulin in Type 2 diabetes. These vaccines, if proven effective, could not only help reduce the need for insulin therapy but may also offer a **preventive measure** for those at high risk of developing diabetes.

Diabetes Vaccines in Development for Type 1 Diabetes

Type 1 diabetes is a condition where the immune system mistakenly attacks and destroys the insulin-producing beta cells of the pancreas. The **underlying cause** of Type 1 diabetes is still not fully understood, but it is believed to involve both **genetic** and **environmental** factors that trigger the immune response.

One of the major goals of **Type 1 diabetes vaccine research** is to **modulate the immune system** and prevent this autoimmune attack on beta cells. This can be achieved through different approaches, primarily focused on either **tolerizing the immune system** or promoting immune responses that protect the beta cells from destruction.

- **Vaccines to Induce Immune Tolerance**: Some experimental vaccines aim to induce **immune tolerance**, essentially retraining the immune system to recognize the body's own insulin-producing cells as "self" and prevent it from attacking them. These vaccines typically consist of **peptides** or **proteins** derived from the beta cells, designed to desensitize the immune system to these targets. By introducing these proteins in a controlled manner, researchers hope to prevent the immune system from attacking the pancreatic beta cells.

- **The DiaPep277 Vaccine**: One of the most promising vaccines in development is the **DiaPep277** vaccine, which is designed to **prevent or delay the onset** of Type 1 diabetes. This vaccine works by targeting the immune system's response to a specific **protein** found in beta cells. By modulating the immune response to this protein, the vaccine aims to slow down or halt the autoimmune attack that destroys insulin-producing cells. Clinical trials have shown some potential in slowing the disease's progression, though more research is needed to determine its effectiveness in long-term use.

- **BHT-3021 Vaccine**: Another notable vaccine candidate is **BHT-3021**, which aims to **prevent beta-cell destruction** by targeting specific immune cells involved in the autoimmune attack. Early-phase trials of BHT-3021 have shown that it may help preserve insulin production in people newly diagnosed with Type 1 diabetes, potentially delaying the need for insulin therapy. However, this vaccine is still in the early stages of development and requires further investigation to assess its safety and efficacy.

- **Combination Therapies**: Some researchers are exploring the idea of combining **vaccines** with other immune-modulating therapies, such as **monoclonal antibodies** or **immune-suppressing drugs**, to enhance their effectiveness in preventing or reversing Type 1 diabetes. The goal is to not only protect beta cells but also promote a healthier immune response overall.

Immune System Modulation in Type 1 Diabetes

The immune system's role in Type 1 diabetes is complex, involving a series of genetic, environmental, and immunological factors that culminate in the destruction of pancreatic beta cells. The process, known as **autoimmunity**, occurs when the body's immune cells mistakenly target its own tissues. In Type 1 diabetes, this involves the immune system targeting the **islets of Langerhans**, which are clusters of cells in the pancreas that include **insulin-producing beta cells**.

The key to developing a vaccine for Type 1 diabetes lies in understanding the mechanisms that trigger this autoimmune response and how they can be **modified** or **halted**. Researchers are focusing on a few main strategies for immune modulation:

- **Antigen-Specific Immunotherapy**: This approach focuses on identifying the specific antigens, or proteins, that are targeted by the immune system in Type 1 diabetes. By using **peptide-based vaccines** or **recombinant proteins**, researchers can develop therapies that specifically target these immune responses, thereby preventing the immune system from attacking the beta cells.

- **Inducing Tolerance to Self-Antigens**: The goal of this strategy is to teach the immune system to tolerate the beta cells. This would involve exposing the immune system to specific **self-antigens**—proteins found in the insulin-producing cells—so that the immune cells no longer recognize them as foreign and attack them. This approach could lead to a **long-lasting** resolution of autoimmune activity, effectively halting the progression of Type 1 diabetes.

- **Regulatory T Cells (Tregs)**: Regulatory T cells play an important role in maintaining immune tolerance. Scientists are investigating whether it is possible to stimulate these Tregs to suppress the autoimmune response in Type 1 diabetes. By promoting the activity of Tregs, it may be possible to prevent the immune system from attacking the beta cells in the pancreas.

<h1 style="text-align:center">Vaccines for Type 2 Diabetes</h1>

While the primary focus of **diabetes vaccine research** has been on Type 1 diabetes, some researchers are also exploring the possibility of vaccines for **Type 2 diabetes**, especially those aimed at improving **insulin sensitivity** and reducing the **risk factors** for the disease. The development of vaccines for **Type 2 diabetes** is more challenging because the underlying mechanisms involve **insulin resistance** rather than autoimmune destruction of beta cells.

- **Immunization Against Insulin Resistance**: Some vaccine research for Type 2 diabetes has focused on the idea of **immunizing against insulin resistance**. The goal here is to modulate the immune system in a way that reduces **chronic inflammation**, a key factor in the development of insulin resistance. By targeting the inflammatory pathways that interfere with insulin signaling, these vaccines may help improve the body's response to insulin and prevent or slow the progression of Type 2 diabetes.

- **Prevention and Early Intervention**: Vaccines may also be used to prevent Type 2 diabetes in people who are at **high risk**, such as those with **pre-diabetes, obesity,** or **a family history** of the disease. The goal of these vaccines would be to prevent the onset of insulin resistance or to slow down the progression of the disease, potentially reducing the need for medications like **metformin** and **insulin**.

<h2 style="text-align:center">Challenges and Future Directions</h2>

While the idea of **vaccines for diabetes** is promising, there are several challenges that need to be addressed before these vaccines can be made widely available:

- **Safety and Efficacy**: Any vaccine developed for diabetes must undergo rigorous testing to ensure that it is both **safe** and **effective**. Since Type 1 diabetes involves an autoimmune process, there is the concern that vaccinating individuals could inadvertently trigger other autoimmune diseases. Therefore, careful monitoring and trials are needed.

- **Long-Term Impact**: Vaccines for Type 1 diabetes will need to demonstrate long-term benefits. It is not enough for a vaccine to simply prevent beta cell destruction in the short term; it must also preserve **insulin production** for years, ideally for a lifetime.

- **Individual Variability**: Given that diabetes is a complex disease with multiple factors at play, the response to a diabetes vaccine may vary from person to person. Researchers will need to understand how **genetic** and **environmental** factors affect the immune response to vaccines in order to tailor therapies for different individuals.

Despite these challenges, the progress made in **diabetes vaccine development** over the past few years is promising. The potential to **prevent** or **modify** the course of diabetes with a vaccine would mark a monumental shift in how we approach the treatment and management of the disease.

Conclusion

The development of **diabetes vaccines** represents one of the most exciting frontiers in medical research. For **Type 1 diabetes**, vaccines that **modulate the immune system** and prevent the autoimmune destruction of beta cells could one day eliminate the need for insulin therapy and offer a potential cure. Similarly, for **Type 2 diabetes**, vaccines designed to improve **insulin sensitivity** or prevent the development of insulin resistance may become a critical tool in managing and preventing the disease.

Although these vaccines are still in the early stages of development, the potential impact they could have on millions of people living with diabetes is immense. As research progresses, we may see a future where diabetes is no longer a chronic disease but a condition that can be prevented, treated, and even cured through **immune system modulation and innovative vaccine technologies**.

Chapter 37

Living with Type 1 Diabetes: Personal Stories

Type 1 diabetes (T1D) is a chronic condition that profoundly affects every aspect of a person's life. While the medical advancements in insulin therapy and monitoring have dramatically improved the outlook for people living with diabetes, the emotional, social, and physical challenges of living with this condition remain ever-present. This chapter shares a collection of **personal stories** from individuals who live with **Type 1 diabetes** and offers insight into their **journey**—their struggles, triumphs, and the ways they navigate daily life while managing a lifelong condition.

These stories highlight the resilience of those living with T1D, as well as the unique challenges they face—both visible and invisible. From the moment of diagnosis to the complexities of day-to-day management, individuals living with **Type 1 diabetes** show us the strength of the human spirit in the face of adversity.

The Emotional Toll of Type 1 Diabetes

Living with Type 1 diabetes is not just about managing **blood sugar levels**; it's about dealing with the constant awareness of one's health and the emotional burden that can come with it. The diagnosis often brings a cascade of emotions, from **fear** and **uncertainty** to feelings of **grief** and **loss**. Individuals with T1D face the overwhelming task of incorporating **insulin therapy**, **blood glucose monitoring**, and constant self-management into their daily routine. This means making thousands of small decisions every day about food, exercise, and insulin use, often with no clear answer for what might work best at any given moment.

For many people, the emotional challenges of living with Type 1 diabetes are compounded by feelings of **isolation**. Unlike Type 2 diabetes, which often develops later in life and is associated with risk factors like obesity or inactivity, Type 1 diabetes is typically diagnosed in childhood or early adulthood. This creates a sense of being "different" at a time when fitting in and being like everyone else feels so important.

One story that stands out is of **Rachel**, diagnosed at age 8. She recalls how, as a young child, she often felt **ashamed** of her condition and kept it hidden from her peers. "It was hard to explain to my friends why I had to leave class to check my blood sugar or why I couldn't always participate in gym class the way they could," Rachel shares. As she grew older, she became more comfortable with her diabetes, but the emotional weight still lingered. "There are days when it feels like diabetes is all I think about. It can be really draining. But over time, I've learned that it's just part of who I am, and I can't let it define me."

The Physical Challenges of Managing Type 1 Diabetes

The physical challenges of living with **Type 1 diabetes** are often the most visible, particularly when it comes to managing blood glucose levels and insulin. Insulin injections, blood sugar tests, and **continuous glucose monitoring** (CGM) devices become constant companions for individuals with T1D. Though advancements in technology have made managing diabetes easier and more accurate, these physical interventions are still a daily necessity.

Many individuals with **Type 1 diabetes** experience fluctuations in blood sugar that can affect energy levels, mood, and physical well-being. **Hypoglycemia** (low blood sugar) and **hyperglycemia** (high blood sugar) are constant threats, and managing them requires vigilance. **Sam**, a college student, shares the struggles of balancing school, work, and life with Type 1 diabetes. "There are days when my blood sugar is all over the place," Sam explains. "I can feel myself getting weak or dizzy from low blood sugar, or sometimes I'm just exhausted from fighting high blood sugars. It's hard to focus when my body feels out of control."

The physical challenges are not just related to blood sugar management. People with Type 1 diabetes are at a higher risk of developing long-term complications like **diabetic neuropathy**, **retinopathy**, and **kidney disease**. The fear of these potential complications is a daily concern for many, including **Liam**, a 45-year-old who was diagnosed with Type 1 diabetes in his twenties. "I'm always thinking about my long-term health. I make sure to get my eye exams, check my feet regularly, and monitor my kidney function. It's a lot, but I know it's necessary to keep the complications at bay," Liam reflects.

The Social and Lifestyle Impacts of Type 1 Diabetes

The social and lifestyle impacts of Type 1 diabetes are profound, as managing the disease requires constant awareness and adaptation to different situations. Social events, family gatherings, work, and school all require careful planning and extra effort. **Emily**, a young professional, describes the challenge of attending social events where food and drink are the focus. "It's always a bit awkward when everyone is having dessert and I have to explain why I can't indulge the same way. I always carry extra supplies with me just in case something goes wrong with my blood sugar, but it feels like I'm always the one who's different," she says. Additionally, living with Type 1 diabetes means individuals must plan their day around food, exercise, and insulin.

James, a 32-year-old lawyer, shares how he balances his busy job with his diabetes management: "I have to plan every meal ahead of time. I'm constantly calculating my insulin dose and adjusting my plans based on how much activity I'll be doing. When I travel for work, I always need to make sure I have my insulin, test strips, and a backup plan in case I get a low blood sugar. It's not just an inconvenience; it's a lifestyle."

The added layer of **stigma** that often accompanies Type 1 diabetes—particularly the assumption that it's caused by lifestyle choices—can be another source of stress. **Olivia**, a teenager diagnosed at age 14, recalls being misunderstood by her peers. "I remember kids telling me that I couldn't have diabetes because I wasn't overweight, or they'd think it was just something I could 'get over.' It made me feel like I had to hide it even more," she says. This social misunderstanding can affect self-esteem and add an emotional burden to the already difficult task of managing the disease.

The Triumphs: Overcoming Obstacles and Finding Hope

Despite these emotional, social, and physical challenges, many individuals with **Type 1 diabetes** find ways to thrive. Whether through **support groups**, **technology**, or personal perseverance, the strength to live a fulfilling life is possible.

Sarah, a marathon runner diagnosed with Type 1 diabetes at 22, exemplifies the power of resilience. "When I first got diagnosed, I thought my athletic career was over. But with careful monitoring, proper insulin management, and a lot of hard work, I've managed to not only keep my blood sugar levels in control but also run marathons. It's possible to live an active life with diabetes—it just takes dedication," Sarah shares. Her story has inspired countless others to pursue their goals and dream big, even in the face of diabetes.

Likewise, many individuals with Type 1 diabetes find solace in **community**. Online forums, local support groups, and social media have made it easier for people with diabetes to connect, share experiences, and offer support. The sense of camaraderie and shared understanding helps individuals feel less isolated and more empowered to manage their condition.

In the case of **David**, a 56-year-old father diagnosed with Type 1 diabetes as a teenager, the support of his family has been crucial. "My kids understand what I go through every day. They know when I need to check my blood sugar or if I need extra help with something. Their understanding makes all the difference. It's not just my fight—it's our fight."

Conclusion: The Journey Continues

The stories shared here reflect the **diverse experiences** of living with **Type 1 diabetes**, from the emotional and social struggles to the physical challenges and personal triumphs. Living with Type 1 diabetes is not an easy journey, but the resilience, courage, and determination of those who face it head-on is nothing short of inspiring. By sharing their stories, individuals with Type 1 diabetes help others feel less alone and offer hope that a fulfilling, active, and rewarding life is still possible despite the constant management the disease requires.

For those who are newly diagnosed or struggling with the complexities of managing diabetes, these stories serve as reminders that **diabetes is not the end of the journey**—it's just a part of the adventure. The strength to live well with diabetes is found in the community, in new medical advancements, and in the hope that, with time, a cure may one day be found.

Chapter 38

Living with Type 2 Diabetes: Personal Stories

Type 2 diabetes (T2D) is a condition that many people live with daily, and its impact on their lives can be both profound and transformative. For some, the diagnosis of Type 2 diabetes is a wake-up call, leading to significant changes in lifestyle, diet, and health management. For others, it may take years before they fully grasp the need to make changes. But regardless of how it begins, the journey of living with **Type 2 diabetes** is a deeply personal one, filled with challenges, learnings, and growth.

This chapter shares the stories of individuals who have been diagnosed with **Type 2 diabetes**, and highlights how they have managed the disease through **lifestyle changes** and **personal transformation**. These real-life stories provide insight into the emotional, social, and physical struggles faced by those with Type 2 diabetes, and they demonstrate the power of **determination** and **self-care** in managing the disease. From making **dietary changes** to incorporating exercise into daily routines, these individuals found ways to take control of their health and improve their quality of life. Their experiences are proof that Type 2 diabetes, while a chronic condition, can be managed—and even reversed—through thoughtful and consistent efforts.

The Moment of Diagnosis: A Turning Point

For many, the moment of being diagnosed with Type 2 diabetes is a turning point in life. The news often comes as a shock, especially for those who feel relatively healthy or who have been living with symptoms without knowing what they meant. **David**, a 48-year-old father of two, recalls the moment he received his diagnosis: "I had been feeling more tired than usual, and I was always thirsty. I didn't think much of it at first, but when my doctor told me I had Type 2 diabetes, it was like a punch to the gut. I thought, 'How could this happen to me? I'm not overweight, and I don't have a family history of diabetes.' But the reality set in quickly, and I knew I had to make some serious changes."

For **Maria**, a 54-year-old teacher, the diagnosis came after years of managing **high blood pressure** and **elevated cholesterol**. "I thought I was doing okay with my health, but when my doctor explained the connection between my other health issues and Type 2 diabetes, it all started to make sense," she says. "I realized that my poor eating habits and lack of exercise were contributing factors. I didn't want to end up with complications like heart disease or kidney failure, so I decided to take action."

The emotional response to a Type 2 diabetes diagnosis is often a mixture of **shock**, **fear**, and **guilt**. People may feel overwhelmed by the idea of having to make lifelong changes to their lifestyle. However, the turning point is often the catalyst for change, prompting individuals to seek solutions and explore ways to improve their health.

Making Lifestyle Changes: A New Beginning

One of the most powerful themes in the stories of people living with Type 2 diabetes is the **transformation through lifestyle changes**. Lifestyle changes are not only the cornerstone of managing Type 2 diabetes—they can also reverse the condition in some individuals, leading to **normalization of blood sugar levels** and a reduction in symptoms. These stories illustrate how important it is to adopt healthier habits, both mentally and physically, to regain control over diabetes.

James, a 60-year-old retired engineer, was diagnosed with Type 2 diabetes after experiencing frequent urination, fatigue, and weight gain. "When I first got diagnosed, I was in denial. I was eating fast food regularly and didn't make time for exercise. But when I saw my blood sugar numbers continuing to rise, I knew something had to change," James explains. "I started by cutting out sugary drinks and junk food. I switched to whole grains, lean proteins, and more vegetables. I also began walking every day for 30 minutes. It wasn't easy at first, but I felt better, and my blood sugar levels started to improve."

For **Samantha**, a 35-year-old marketing manager, her journey began with the realization that she had been ignoring the signs of Type 2 diabetes for years. "I was always exhausted, and I was gaining weight. I had been under a lot of stress at work and just didn't pay attention to my health. When my doctor told me I was prediabetic, I knew I had to change my habits before I developed full-blown diabetes."

Samantha decided to overhaul her diet by cutting out processed foods and focusing on **whole, nutrient-dense meals**. "I started preparing my own meals and making sure they were balanced. I also started doing yoga and strength training three times a week," she says. Within months, Samantha saw remarkable improvements not only in her blood sugar levels but also in her **energy levels** and overall well-being.

Adopting these lifestyle changes isn't always easy, but it's possible with patience, consistency, and support from loved ones. **Helen**, a 45-year-old nurse, struggled with **obesity** and was diagnosed with Type 2 diabetes after years of an unhealthy diet and lack of physical activity. "It was a wake-up call," she recalls. "I knew I had to make changes if I didn't want to end up in the hospital with complications." Helen lost over 60 pounds by changing her diet and increasing her physical activity, incorporating both **cardio** and **strength training** into her routine. "I focus on eating lean proteins, healthy fats, and plenty of vegetables. It wasn't an overnight change, but over time I started feeling stronger and more in control."

The Power of Support and Education

For many individuals living with Type 2 diabetes, having a strong support system is key to staying motivated and on track. Support from family members, friends, and even online communities can provide both emotional and practical guidance during difficult times.

Daniel, a 41-year-old software developer, acknowledges how important it was to have his family's support as he changed his lifestyle. "When I was diagnosed, I felt like I was in this alone. But my wife and kids were incredibly supportive. They helped me prepare meals and made sure we were all eating healthier. We started exercising together as a family, and it became a fun way to bond," Daniel shares.

Education also plays a critical role in managing Type 2 diabetes. Many individuals benefit from learning about their condition and understanding how their lifestyle affects their blood sugar levels.

Leah, a 52-year-old administrative assistant, took a diabetes education class at her local clinic. "It was a game-changer," she explains. "I learned about portion control, reading food labels, and the importance of balanced meals. The class gave me the tools I needed to make smart decisions about my health." By using what she learned in class, Leah was able to bring her blood sugar levels under control and lose weight in a healthy way. "I no longer feel like I'm guessing with my food choices. I know what works for my body, and I'm committed to staying on track."

Overcoming Obstacles: Persistence and Mindset

Though lifestyle changes can be transformative, living with Type 2 diabetes often means facing obstacles along the way. The journey to better health is rarely linear, and setbacks are a normal part of the process. Many individuals experience **difficult days** when motivation wanes or life circumstances create barriers to staying on track.

Christopher, a 50-year-old teacher, had a breakthrough moment when he realized that, while lifestyle changes were crucial, his mindset needed to shift as well. "I was doing everything right—eating healthy and exercising regularly—but I kept thinking of diabetes as a burden. I felt like I was constantly fighting against it," Christopher admits. "It wasn't until I started seeing my condition as something I could manage, rather than something that defined me, that I truly felt empowered." By embracing a positive mindset and acknowledging his progress, Christopher learned to navigate the challenges of living with Type 2 diabetes more effectively.

Barbara, a 59-year-old accountant, recalls the times she felt frustrated when her blood sugar levels weren't where she wanted them to be. "It's easy to get discouraged when you don't see immediate results, but I had to remind myself that this is a marathon, not a sprint. Managing diabetes is about consistency, not perfection." By embracing this mindset, Barbara has learned to **celebrate small victories** and continue making progress, even when things don't go according to plan.

Living Fully with Type 2 Diabetes

The stories shared in this chapter reflect the strength and resilience of individuals living with Type 2 diabetes. While the condition presents challenges, it also offers an opportunity for growth and transformation. By making lifestyle changes and committing to self-care, individuals can **regain control** over their health, reduce their symptoms, and live full, active lives.

As **Steven**, a 44-year-old small business owner, puts it: "Diabetes doesn't define me, but it has changed my life for the better. I'm healthier now than I was 10 years ago, and I'm not just surviving—I'm thriving. It's all about taking small steps and making choices that work for me."

These personal stories illustrate that **Type 2 diabetes** is a manageable condition, and with the right mindset, support, and lifestyle changes, anyone with the condition can lead a fulfilling, vibrant life.

Chapter 39

Overcoming the Emotional Impact of Diabetes

Diabetes is often referred to as a "silent" disease, but its emotional impact can be anything but quiet. For those living with diabetes, especially over long periods of time, the constant management of blood sugar levels, medication regimens, and lifestyle adjustments can take a toll on mental health. While diabetes is a physical disease, its emotional consequences—such as stress, anxiety, depression, and **diabetes distress**—are just as real and significant.

The emotional weight can sometimes feel as burdensome as the physical symptoms of the disease.   However, many individuals with diabetes have found ways to cope with, and even thrive despite, the challenges that come with the condition. This chapter explores stories of **resilience, hope**, and **success** in managing not only the physical aspects of diabetes but also its emotional toll.

The Unseen Struggles: Living with the Emotional Burden of Diabetes

When people are diagnosed with diabetes, especially Type 1 or Type 2, they may find themselves navigating a complex array of emotions. Initially, there is often a sense of shock or disbelief, followed by fear of what the future might hold. The emotional burden can be further complicated by **diabetes-related complications**, such as neuropathy, retinopathy, and cardiovascular disease. **Sarah**, a 30-year-old woman with Type 1 diabetes, remembers feeling overwhelmed when she was first diagnosed: "I didn't know what diabetes would mean for me long-term. I felt like I had to be perfect all the time, constantly watching my blood sugar and worrying about complications."

For **Carlos**, a 52-year-old man with Type 2 diabetes, the emotional toll was profound. "At first, I thought I could just take medication and keep living my life the same way. But the reality is, diabetes requires constant attention—meal planning, monitoring blood sugar, exercise. It felt exhausting and isolating. I was afraid of what would happen if I didn't keep up with everything," Carlos admits.

These feelings of stress and fear are common among people newly diagnosed with diabetes. As the disease progresses and the necessity for constant management becomes more pronounced, **diabetes distress** can creep in. Unlike the physical symptoms, which may be visible or quantifiable, **emotional distress** often goes unrecognized or misunderstood, leaving individuals to face their struggles alone.

Resilience in the Face of Diabetes Distress

While the emotional toll of diabetes is significant, many people who live with the disease find ways to turn their struggles into strength. **Resilience** is a core theme that runs through many personal stories of people managing diabetes. For some, the journey involves acknowledging the emotional weight of the disease and finding coping mechanisms to manage it. For others, resilience comes from the gradual realization that living with diabetes doesn't mean being defined by it.

Tara, a 41-year-old mother of three with Type 2 diabetes, struggled with **depression** early in her diagnosis. "I was overwhelmed by the constant worry about my blood sugar levels. I would test my blood sugar multiple times a day, and it was a constant cycle of anxiety," she shares.

"There were days when I felt like I couldn't keep up with everything—parenting, working, managing diabetes."

However, over time, Tara found ways to build resilience. "I started attending support groups for people with diabetes, which really helped me connect with others who understood what I was going through. I also started practicing mindfulness and meditation, which helped me manage stress. I learned to not just focus on the numbers but on how I felt overall. I began to see the whole picture—managing my diabetes and my emotional health was just as important." Tara's story highlights the critical role of **support systems** and **self-care** practices in managing the emotional impact of diabetes.

Hope Through Action: Transforming Diabetes into a Source of Empowerment

For many, hope comes from the knowledge that **positive changes**—whether through lifestyle adjustments, mental health support, or a shift in mindset—can significantly improve both their emotional and physical well-being. **John**, a 58-year-old man living with Type 2 diabetes, found hope through **education** and **action**. "I used to feel like I was constantly battling my body. I didn't understand how my choices affected my blood sugar. Once I educated myself and learned about proper nutrition, exercise, and how to monitor my blood sugar effectively, I felt more in control," John says.

Over time, John began to embrace his diagnosis as a way to take control of his health rather than letting it control him. "I started small—walking every day, cutting out sugary snacks, and learning to cook healthier meals. I didn't expect overnight changes, but every small victory helped me feel more hopeful about my future."

The emotional turnaround came when John realized that he wasn't powerless in the face of diabetes. "It was a huge mental shift. I went from feeling like I was fighting against my body to understanding that I could work with my body. Managing diabetes became a source of empowerment."

The Role of Support and Community: Reaching Out for Help

Support is often essential for overcoming the emotional challenges of living with diabetes. Many individuals find strength in their relationships with family, friends, healthcare providers, and peer support groups.

Emily, a 45-year-old teacher with Type 1 diabetes, recalls the importance of seeking help: "I used to try to deal with everything on my own. But I quickly realized that having a support system made a huge difference in my emotional well-being. My husband has been my rock, and I also found a community of other women with Type 1 diabetes who truly understand the unique struggles."

Support groups—whether in-person or online—offer a safe space where individuals can share their struggles, exchange advice, and offer encouragement. This shared understanding can help alleviate feelings of isolation, making it easier to manage the emotional burden of diabetes.

David, who was diagnosed with Type 2 diabetes at age 48, found solace in an online community dedicated to managing the condition. "I started following diabetes blogs and joining online forums. It was comforting to hear from others who were going through the same thing. I realized I wasn't alone in this journey."

Healthcare professionals also play an important role in addressing the emotional challenges of diabetes. By fostering open communication and providing psychological support, doctors, diabetes educators, and counselors can help individuals cope with **diabetes distress** and address underlying mental health concerns, such as **depression** and **anxiety**.

Mindfulness and Mental Health: Addressing the Psychological Impact of Diabetes

As the research into diabetes care evolves, there is increasing recognition of the need for **mental health care** alongside physical treatment. Studies have shown that individuals with diabetes are at a higher risk for developing mental health conditions such as **depression**, **anxiety**, and **diabetes distress**.

Carlos, who struggled with **mental health issues** after his diagnosis, sought help through therapy and medication. "I didn't realize how much the emotional aspect of diabetes was affecting me. It wasn't just the physical side that was challenging—it was the fear, the uncertainty, the feeling that I couldn't keep up. I eventually started seeing a therapist, and that really helped me put everything in perspective. I learned coping strategies to manage stress and anxiety, which helped me feel more at peace with my diabetes."

In addition to traditional mental health support, **mindfulness** and **cognitive behavioral therapy (CBT)** have been shown to be effective in helping individuals manage the emotional side of diabetes. **Mindfulness** involves being present in the moment, reducing stress, and cultivating a positive mindset. **CBT** helps individuals identify and change negative thought patterns that contribute to emotional distress, teaching them healthier ways of thinking and coping.

Living with diabetes is undoubtedly challenging, but it is possible to overcome the emotional struggles that accompany the disease. Whether through **education**, **support systems**, **mental health care**, or **lifestyle changes**, individuals can find ways to live fulfilling lives despite the challenges. The stories shared in this chapter illustrate the power of resilience, hope, and self-care in managing the emotional impact of diabetes.

As **Tara** puts it, "Diabetes doesn't define who I am. It's a part of my life, but it's not my whole life. I've learned to live with it and not let it control me. It's about taking one day at a time and being kind to myself." The key takeaway from these stories is that, while the emotional impact of diabetes can be overwhelming at times, it can also be managed with the right tools, mindset, and support. By focusing on **hope**, **empowerment**, and **resilience**, individuals can navigate the emotional complexities of diabetes and build lives that are not only healthier but also filled with joy and purpose.

Chapter 40

The Future of Diabetes Care

Diabetes care has come a long way in recent decades, and the future holds even greater promise. With advancements in **medical research, technology**, and a deeper understanding of the disease, the trajectory of diabetes treatment and management is poised for significant breakthroughs. This chapter will explore the emerging trends and innovations in diabetes care, from cutting-edge therapies to potential cures, and look ahead to the future of diabetes management, emphasizing the importance of continued research and the evolving role of personalized care.

The Promise of Precision Medicine

One of the most exciting directions in the future of diabetes care is the rise of **precision medicine**—an approach that tailor's treatment to the individual based on their genetic makeup, lifestyle, and environmental factors. **Genomic research** has already made significant strides in identifying specific genes that contribute to the development of Type 1 and Type 2 diabetes. As our understanding of the **genetic predispositions** to diabetes deepens, healthcare providers will be able to offer **personalized treatment plans** that target the unique characteristics of each patient's condition.

Precision medicine involves not only genetic testing but also a closer look at how environmental factors, such as diet, stress, and physical activity, interact with a person's genes to influence diabetes risk and management. In the future, genetic testing could become routine for both

early detection of diabetes and for **tailoring treatments** such as medications and lifestyle interventions. This personalized approach holds the potential to improve outcomes and reduce the risk of complications by focusing on the specific needs of each patient, rather than using a one-size-fits-all strategy.

Stem Cell Therapy: A Potential Cure for Type 1 Diabetes

One of the most promising avenues of research is the exploration of **stem cell therapy** as a potential cure for **Type 1 diabetes**. Type 1 diabetes is caused by an autoimmune attack on the insulin-producing beta cells of the pancreas. The ability to regenerate or replace these beta cells using **stem cell therapy** could fundamentally change the treatment landscape for Type 1 diabetes.

Research in this area is still in its early stages, but there have been significant breakthroughs in growing insulin-producing cells from stem cells. Clinical trials are underway to test whether these **beta cell replacements** can function effectively in the human body, potentially eliminating the need for daily insulin injections. Although there is still a long way to go before stem cell treatments become a mainstream therapy for diabetes, the progress made so far provides hope for those with Type 1 diabetes, offering a glimpse of a future where insulin dependency may be a thing of the past.

The Artificial Pancreas: A Leap Toward Better Blood Sugar Control

In the realm of diabetes technology, one of the most revolutionary innovations is the development of the **artificial pancreas**, a system that mimics the function of a healthy pancreas by automatically monitoring blood glucose levels and administering insulin as needed. The artificial pancreas combines **continuous glucose monitoring (CGM)** with an **insulin pump** to regulate blood sugar levels in real time.

Recent advancements have made this technology more sophisticated and accessible, with systems that can even predict blood sugar fluctuations based on data from CGMs. This closed-loop system offers the potential for more precise and stable blood sugar control, reducing the risk of both **hypoglycemia** (low blood sugar) and **hyperglycemia** (high blood sugar), which are common concerns for individuals with Type 1 and Type 2 diabetes. As this technology evolves, it could make diabetes management much simpler and less time-consuming, offering a better quality of life for people with diabetes.

The future of the artificial pancreas also includes integration with other health technologies, such as **smartwatches** and **mobile apps**, to provide real-time insights into diabetes management. As these systems become more refined, individuals with diabetes may have access to a seamless, fully automated approach to blood sugar control.

Smart Insulin: The Next Step in Insulin Therapy

A major breakthrough in the pipeline for diabetes treatment is the development of **smart insulin**—insulin that automatically adjusts based on blood sugar levels. Traditional insulin therapy requires careful management and the understanding of how much insulin is needed at specific times, based on diet, exercise, and other factors. Smart insulin, however, could be designed to activate only when blood sugar levels rise above a certain threshold, automatically releasing insulin in response to higher glucose levels.

This type of insulin would not only make managing Type 1 and Type 2 diabetes easier but could also reduce the risk of dangerous fluctuations in blood sugar levels. Researchers are currently working on creating insulin that is sensitive to glucose, providing a more **dynamic and responsive** way to manage diabetes, potentially reducing the need for frequent monitoring and injections.

The Role of the Gut Microbiome in Diabetes

An emerging area of research in diabetes care is the role of the **gut microbiome**—the community of bacteria and other microorganisms that live in the digestive tract. Studies have shown that the microbiome plays a crucial role in metabolism, immune function, and even insulin sensitivity. Disruptions in the microbiome may contribute to the development of **insulin resistance** in Type 2 diabetes.

Researchers are now investigating ways to influence the gut microbiome to improve diabetes outcomes. This may include the use of **probiotics**, **prebiotics**, or **fecal microbiota transplants (FMT)** to restore a healthy balance of bacteria in the gut. Early studies suggest that modifying the microbiome could improve glucose metabolism and insulin sensitivity, providing a new avenue for diabetes treatment. Additionally, **dietary interventions** designed to support a healthy microbiome are gaining attention. The focus on fiber-rich foods, fermented foods, and other gut-friendly nutrients could play a significant role in preventing and managing diabetes.

Diabetes Vaccines: A New Frontier in Prevention

Another promising area of diabetes research involves the development of **vaccines** aimed at preventing or even treating diabetes. For Type 1 diabetes, research is focused on **immune system modulation** to prevent the autoimmune attack on beta cells that causes the disease. **Vaccine-based therapies** are being studied that could either prevent the onset of Type 1 diabetes in those at risk or, in the future, slow or halt the progression of the disease once diagnosed.

For Type 2 diabetes, vaccine development is more focused on the prevention of **insulin resistance**. Researchers are exploring how vaccines could reduce the body's inflammatory response, which plays a significant role in the development of insulin resistance, a hallmark of Type 2 diabetes. While these vaccines are still in the experimental stage, the potential to prevent diabetes before it develops could revolutionize the way we think about managing and preventing the disease.

Improving Access to Diabetes Care

The future of diabetes care is not just about **advanced therapies** and **cutting-edge technologies**—it's also about improving **access** to care for people around the world. As the global prevalence of diabetes continues to rise, it is crucial to address the healthcare disparities that exist, particularly in underserved and low-income populations. The future of diabetes care must include affordable access to **medications, diagnostic tools**, and **education**.

Technological advancements such as mobile health apps, telemedicine, and remote monitoring could help bridge the gap in access to quality care, especially in rural and low-income areas. These tools have the potential to connect patients with healthcare professionals and offer real-time monitoring and guidance, making it easier for people with diabetes to manage their condition effectively, no matter where they live.

Prevention will continue to play a crucial role in the future of diabetes care. With the rise in **Type 2 diabetes** and **pre-diabetes** diagnoses, public health campaigns aimed at **reducing risk factors** such as **obesity**, **sedentary lifestyles**, and **poor diets** are critical. Education on **healthy eating**, **physical activity**, and **weight management** will remain central to the prevention of Type 2 diabetes.

In the future, targeted interventions at the community level—focused on improving access to nutritious food, exercise facilities, and healthcare—could help slow the rise of diabetes globally. By integrating **prevention** and **early intervention** into public health policy, we could see a decline in the number of new diabetes cases and an overall improvement in the management of the disease.

Conclusion

The future of diabetes care is incredibly exciting, with many advances on the horizon. From **precision medicine** to **stem cell therapies** and **artificial pancreas systems**, the next few decades could bring transformative changes in how we understand, treat, and prevent diabetes. However, these advancements depend on continued research, innovation, and collaboration across the healthcare industry, as well as a commitment to improving access to care for everyone.

As the global diabetes epidemic continues to grow, so too does our knowledge of the disease and our ability to manage it effectively. While there is still much work to be done, the future holds great promise for those living with diabetes, offering hope for better outcomes, improved quality of life, and, ultimately, a potential cure. The journey toward a world without diabetes is well underway, and with each new discovery, we are one step closer to turning that vision into reality.

Chapter 41

Advocacy and Diabetes Awareness

Diabetes is a chronic disease that affects millions of people worldwide, and its global impact continues to grow. As the prevalence of diabetes rises, so too does the need for awareness, education, and advocacy. Raising awareness about diabetes, supporting those affected by it, and advocating for better policies, research funding, and healthcare access are critical for improving outcomes for individuals with diabetes and preventing the further spread of the disease. In this chapter, we will explore how you can become involved in diabetes advocacy, education, and awareness efforts to make a positive difference in the lives of those impacted by diabetes.

The Importance of Diabetes Advocacy

Diabetes advocacy plays a crucial role in addressing the needs of people living with the condition, promoting early detection, and fostering policies that support **diabetes research**, **healthcare access**, and **preventive care**. Advocacy efforts can help raise public awareness about the challenges individuals with diabetes face, reduce stigma, and promote positive changes in healthcare practices, policy development, and funding priorities. Advocating for diabetes can also lead to significant improvements in **health outcomes**, as increased awareness often translates into better access to care, better education, and more research dollars for innovative treatments and potential cures.

In addition to improving healthcare, **advocacy** helps challenge societal barriers that contribute to the diabetes epidemic, such as poor nutrition, lack of physical activity, and limited access to healthcare. Through advocacy, communities can become more aware of the lifestyle choices and environmental factors that contribute to diabetes, leading to more sustainable, long-term changes at both the individual and systemic levels.

Getting Involved in Diabetes Advocacy

There are many ways to become actively involved in **diabetes advocacy**. Whether you are someone living with diabetes, a healthcare professional, a caregiver, or someone who is passionate about public health, your voice can make a significant impact in raising awareness and improving the lives of people with diabetes. Some of the most effective ways to get involved in advocacy include:

Joining Diabetes Advocacy Organizations

There are many **non-profit organizations** and **advocacy groups** focused on diabetes awareness and support. These organizations often provide platforms for people to engage in advocacy efforts, such as lobbying for policy changes, organizing awareness campaigns, and fundraising for diabetes research. Some of the well-known organizations include the **American Diabetes Association (ADA), JDRF (Juvenile Diabetes Research Foundation)**, and the **Diabetes Foundation**. By joining these organizations, you can stay informed about the latest developments in diabetes research, participate in advocacy campaigns, and become part of a larger community dedicated to making a difference.

Advocating for Diabetes Research and Funding:

Research into diabetes, including studies on **preventive strategies, better treatments**, and **potential cures**, is vital to reducing the impact of the disease on individuals and society. Advocating for increased **research funding** is one of the most impactful ways you can contribute to diabetes advocacy. By engaging with policymakers, writing letters, attending advocacy events, and participating in grassroots campaigns, you can help raise awareness about the need for continued investment in **diabetes research**. **Fostering partnerships** between healthcare institutions, governments, and private organizations is essential to ensure that diabetes research remains a priority on national and international agendas.

Raising Public Awareness through Education

Education is one of the most powerful tools in combating diabetes. By raising awareness about the causes, risks, and potential complications of diabetes, we can encourage people to make healthier choices and take proactive steps to prevent or manage the disease. Whether through social media platforms, local events, or public speaking engagements, there are numerous ways to educate the public about diabetes and its impact.

Sharing accurate and up-to-date information about diabetes prevention, symptoms, and management strategies can help reduce misconceptions and empower individuals to take charge of their health. In addition, creating and distributing **educational materials**—such as pamphlets, flyers, and online resources—can help people with diabetes better understand their condition and make informed decisions about their treatment and lifestyle. Schools, workplaces, and community centers are ideal places to distribute educational resources and host informational sessions on diabetes.

Advocacy isn't limited to grassroots efforts; influencing **policy** at local, state, and national levels is another powerful way to address the challenges of diabetes. Engaging with lawmakers and policy decision-makers can result in critical changes, such as increased funding for diabetes research, improved healthcare policies for people with diabetes, and better access to necessary medications and treatment options.

Advocacy efforts at the policy level may include lobbying for laws that support **diabetes management**, **health insurance coverage** for diabetes medications and devices, and **affordable access** to healthy food and exercise programs. Working with policymakers to create **public health initiatives** that focus on **diabetes prevention**, particularly for at-risk populations, can have long-lasting benefits for communities as a whole.

Another aspect of policy advocacy involves pushing for **access to diabetes care** in underserved or marginalized communities. People living in rural or economically disadvantaged areas often face barriers to receiving the healthcare they need, and advocating for equitable healthcare policies can help bridge these gaps.

Fundraising for Diabetes Research and Support

One of the most impactful ways to contribute to the diabetes cause is through **fundraising**. Fundraising efforts directly support diabetes research, patient programs, and community outreach initiatives. Whether through hosting charity events, participating in **walks or runs** organized by diabetes foundations, or launching crowdfunding campaigns, fundraising helps to generate the financial resources needed to make a tangible impact on the fight against diabetes.

Many diabetes organizations offer opportunities for individuals to participate in **fundraising challenges**, such as the **Step Out: Walk to Stop Diabetes** campaign or **JDRF One Walk**, where participants raise money while engaging in physical activity. Corporate sponsorships, community partnerships, and individual donations are all essential in helping fund crucial research and provide educational resources to individuals living with diabetes.

Supporting People with Diabetes: Peer Support and Advocacy

Beyond advocacy and research, another critical aspect of diabetes advocacy is offering **peer support** to individuals living with the disease. Connecting with others who understand the challenges of managing diabetes can provide emotional relief and practical advice. Peer support programs, both online and in person, allow individuals to share their experiences, ask questions, and provide encouragement to one another.

There are also **support groups** for specific groups of people with diabetes, such as **parents of children with Type 1 diabetes, caregivers**, and those diagnosed with **Type 2 diabetes**. These groups offer a safe space for discussing the unique emotional, social, and practical challenges that come with managing diabetes.

Being a **peer advocate** involves using your personal experience with diabetes to support others, raise awareness, and help individuals feel less isolated. It can be as simple as sharing your story with others, volunteering for diabetes-related events, or mentoring newly diagnosed individuals through their journey with the disease.

In today's digital age, social media is a powerful tool for **spreading awareness**, **sharing resources**, and **mobilizing support** for diabetes causes. Platforms like Facebook, Instagram, Twitter, and TikTok offer vast audiences to advocate for diabetes care, education, and research. Digital advocacy allows people from all walks of life to share their stories, connect with others, and participate in global movements.

Organizations like the **American Diabetes Association** and **JDRF** frequently utilize social media to host awareness campaigns, engage with supporters, and promote diabetes-related events. Social media campaigns such as **#DiabetesAwarenessMonth** or **#Type1DiabetesAwareness** provide a unique opportunity to spread knowledge and rally individuals and groups around a common cause.

By sharing articles, personal stories, and updates on diabetes-related news, you can contribute to the ongoing conversation and help reduce the stigma surrounding the disease. Many individuals with diabetes also use **Instagram** or **YouTube** to document their journeys and offer advice to others, creating a **virtual support network** that extends far beyond local communities.

Conclusion

The future of diabetes care, research, and prevention is largely shaped by **advocacy**. Whether through raising awareness, supporting research, improving healthcare access, or advocating for policy changes, everyone has a role to play in tackling the diabetes epidemic. By becoming actively involved in advocacy efforts, you not only help to improve the lives of those currently living with diabetes but also contribute to a world where

prevention, **early diagnosis**, and **better management** of diabetes are universally accessible.

Diabetes awareness and advocacy efforts are integral to changing public attitudes, reducing the burden of the disease on healthcare systems, and empowering individuals to take control of their health. Whether you're **participating in awareness campaigns**, **fundraising**, or simply **sharing information**, your involvement can make a real difference.

Through continued **education**, **empowerment**, and **collaboration**, we can work together to ensure that diabetes no longer has to define lives, and that those who live with it are given the resources, care, and support they need to thrive.

Chapter 42

How to Build a Support Network

Managing diabetes can be an overwhelming journey, both physically and emotionally. While living with diabetes requires commitment to self-care, regular monitoring, and making daily decisions about diet and activity, the process doesn't have to be faced alone. Building a **support network** is one of the most important steps individuals with diabetes can take to manage their condition effectively and thrive despite the challenges. A strong support network can provide **emotional encouragement, practical advice**, and a sense of community, all of which are vital in reducing stress and improving overall well-being.

In this chapter, we will explore the **importance of family, friends, healthcare providers**, and **online communities** in building a robust support system. We will discuss how each of these elements can help manage diabetes more effectively, improve health outcomes, and provide a sense of connection and solidarity in the face of a chronic illness.

The Role of Family in Diabetes Support

For many people with diabetes, family is the cornerstone of their support network. A supportive family can have a profound effect on an individual's ability to manage their condition and feel empowered in their daily life. Family members can provide emotional support, encouragement, and help with **practical tasks** such as meal planning, monitoring blood sugar levels, or attending medical appointments.

Understanding and Communication

One of the most important factors in involving family in diabetes care is open communication. It's essential for family members to have a clear understanding of the diagnosis and how the condition affects their loved one's life. This includes not only the physical aspects, such as managing blood sugar levels and taking medications, but also the emotional and psychological impact that diabetes can have. Family members who are well-informed about the condition can offer better support, be more empathetic to the challenges, and assist in ways that contribute to better management of diabetes.

Involving family in diabetes education can help reduce feelings of isolation for the person with diabetes. When family members understand the importance of **healthy eating, physical activity**, and **consistent monitoring**, they can better support lifestyle changes and even make these changes as a family. Additionally, the family can be a key player in creating a positive home environment that encourages self-care without enabling unhealthy habits.

Emotional Support

Diabetes is not just a medical condition; it's a chronic condition that can affect a person's emotional health. Family members who offer emotional support can help mitigate feelings of **frustration, anxiety**, and **depression**, which are common among people with diabetes. Whether through **listening**, offering encouragement, or helping with stress management, family members can provide a vital emotional anchor. Having a family member to talk to when things are difficult or when challenges arise can make a huge difference. **Social support** from loved ones has been shown to improve diabetes outcomes, as it can reduce stress and enhance **self-management skills**.

The Role of Friends in Diabetes Support

While family members are often the first line of defense, friends also play an essential role in the **social and emotional** aspects of living with diabetes. **Close friends** can provide a level of companionship and understanding that may not be possible in family relationships. They can help people with diabetes feel less isolated and more connected to the world around them.

Peer Support

Friends who understand or are willing to learn about diabetes can be a crucial support source. They may be more empathetic because they are not as emotionally involved as family members, but they still provide a sense of belonging. A **trusted friend** can offer advice, share personal experiences, and engage in activities that support **diabetes management**, such as attending **exercise classes** together or cooking healthy meals.

Friends can also be a great source of emotional **relief**. Sometimes, the burden of managing a chronic illness can be overwhelming, and having a nonjudgmental, supportive friend to talk to can relieve some of the stress and anxiety. Good friends can remind individuals with diabetes to take care of themselves and encourage them to seek help when needed.

Building a Social Circle of Supportive Friends

Building a circle of **supportive friends** who understand the challenges of living with diabetes can be invaluable. These friends can be a positive influence, helping to encourage self-care behaviors and reducing the sense of isolation that often accompanies chronic illness. Socializing in a supportive environment can foster mental well-being and emotional resilience, key components of effective diabetes management.

While family and friends play a critical role in providing emotional support and practical help, healthcare providers are the **cornerstone** of effective **diabetes management**. These professionals provide the technical expertise, guidance, and medical supervision necessary to manage the disease and avoid complications.

Building a Collaborative Relationship with Your Doctor open, communicative relationship with a healthcare provider is essential for successful diabetes management. Your doctor should be viewed as a **partner** in your care, someone you trust and work with to monitor blood sugar levels, adjust medications, and create a plan for managing your condition. Many people with diabetes benefit from **team-based care**, where a primary care physician, endocrinologist, diabetes educator, dietitian, and mental health professional all work together to create an individualized care plan.

A positive relationship with your healthcare team encourages collaboration. You should feel comfortable discussing your concerns, symptoms, and treatment options with them. **Regular check-ups** and blood tests are crucial in preventing complications and monitoring the progression of diabetes. Your doctor will not only track your blood sugar levels but also ensure that your cholesterol, kidney function, and overall health are being well-managed.

Diabetes Educators and Specialists

Certified diabetes educators (CDEs) are healthcare professionals who specialize in teaching individuals with diabetes how to manage their condition effectively. They can help with everything from meal planning and exercise guidance to understanding medication regimens and

emotional coping strategies. Building a relationship with a diabetes educator can be a valuable resource for acquiring in-depth knowledge about managing diabetes on a daily basis.

If you're living with diabetes, don't hesitate to ask for referrals to specialists, such as an **endocrinologist**, **nephrologist**, or **ophthalmologist**, to monitor the specific areas of health that diabetes can impact.

The Importance of Online Communities and Peer Support Groups

In addition to the **in-person** support provided by family, friends, and healthcare professionals, online communities have become a vital resource for people living with diabetes. The ability to connect with others who share similar experiences, challenges, and successes can be incredibly empowering and comforting.

Online Support Groups

There are countless **online communities** and **support groups** dedicated to diabetes, ranging from Facebook groups to forums on health websites like Diabetes.co.uk and My Diabetes Home. These spaces allow individuals to ask questions, share personal experiences, and get advice from people who truly understand what they're going through. Whether you're newly diagnosed or have been living with diabetes for years, online communities offer a wealth of **emotional support** and practical insights.

The Power of Shared Experiences

One of the greatest benefits of online communities is the opportunity to connect with people who are in similar circumstances. Whether you're struggling with the emotional burden of diabetes or need advice on managing blood sugar levels, others in these communities can offer firsthand experiences and coping strategies. In these online spaces, there's a sense of shared responsibility to support one another and celebrate victories, no matter how small.

Online support groups also allow for anonymity and privacy, which can be appealing to those who feel uncomfortable discussing their condition in person. You can learn from others, share your successes, and even **find new friends** who share your interest in managing diabetes together.

Mental Health Professionals: Emotional Support for Diabetes Management

Managing a chronic condition like diabetes can take a toll on mental health, and sometimes the emotional burden requires professional assistance. **Mental health professionals**, including therapists and counselors, can help individuals cope with the emotional complexities of living with diabetes, such as **diabetes distress**, **depression**, or **anxiety**. A mental health professional can work with individuals to build **stress management** techniques, **coping strategies**, and address any **mental health concerns** that may impact their ability to effectively manage their condition. This support is essential in building resilience, improving quality of life, and ensuring that diabetes does not unduly interfere with personal well-being.

Conclusion

Living with diabetes can be challenging, but it is important to remember that you do not have to navigate this journey alone. By building a comprehensive support network of **family, friends, healthcare providers**, and **online communities**, you can ensure that you have the resources, encouragement, and guidance needed to manage your condition successfully.

The power of a strong support network lies in its ability to provide both **emotional resilience** and **practical assistance**. It helps individuals with diabetes feel empowered, less isolated, and better able to manage the day-to-day challenges that come with living with a chronic condition. The support you receive, both in person and online, can play a pivotal role in ensuring that you live a fulfilling and healthy life, regardless of your diagnosis.

By leaning on others for support and offering support in return, you contribute to creating a **strong, compassionate community** where diabetes is not just a personal journey, but a shared experience. Through this connection, you can **manage your diabetes more effectively**, overcome emotional hurdles, and thrive.

Chapter 43

A Comprehensive Diabetes Toolkit

Living with diabetes requires more than just medical care and lifestyle adjustments—it involves constant learning, staying updated on new research, and having the right resources at your fingertips. From tracking your blood sugar levels to managing your diet and emotional well-being, there are countless tools, apps, books, and websites that can support and guide you throughout your diabetes journey.

This **Comprehensive Diabetes Toolkit** serves as a one-stop collection of the best resources, educational materials, and support networks to help you manage your diabetes more effectively. Whether you're newly diagnosed or have been living with diabetes for years, these resources will equip you with the knowledge, skills, and support you need to thrive.

Apps for Diabetes Management

Technology has revolutionized the way we manage health, and **diabetes apps** are some of the most powerful tools for tracking glucose levels, medication, meals, and physical activity. These apps not only help you stay organized but also provide insights into your blood sugar trends, which are essential for adjusting your lifestyle and treatment plan.

Glucose Tracking Apps

Apps like **MySugar**, **Carb Manager**, and **BlueLoop** are designed specifically for tracking blood sugar levels and providing reports that can be shared with your healthcare provider. These apps allow you to log your glucose readings, insulin doses, meals, and exercise routines, making it easier to spot patterns and manage your diabetes more effectively.

Meal Planning and Carb Counting Apps

For people with diabetes, understanding food and its impact on blood sugar is essential. Apps like **Carb Manager**, **MyFitnessPal**, and **Fooducate** help users keep track of their meals, count carbohydrates, and understand the nutritional value of different foods. These apps offer barcode scanners, preloaded food databases, and even custom meal planning options to help individuals stay on top of their daily nutrition.

Exercise Tracking Apps

Physical activity is a key component of diabetes management. Apps like **Fitbit**, **Google Fit**, and **Strava** help you monitor your daily steps, exercise routines, and overall physical activity. These apps can also be integrated with glucose tracking apps to give a complete picture of how exercise affects your blood sugar, which can guide better lifestyle choices.

Diabetes Management and Education Apps

There are also several apps designed to provide education, resources, and support, such as **Glucose Buddy** and **Diabetes Connect**. These apps help you track glucose levels, medications, and health records while also offering useful tips and resources about diabetes self-management. Some apps even include daily reminders for medications, glucose testing, and hydration, so you can stay on top of your daily diabetes care routine.

Books for Diabetes Education

Books are invaluable resources for gaining in-depth knowledge about diabetes and learning how to manage the condition from a scientific and practical standpoint. Whether you're looking for tips on controlling blood sugar, recipes for managing your diet, or personal stories of others living with diabetes, there are many books available that can enhance your understanding and provide encouragement.

The Diabetes Code by Dr. Jason Fung

Dr. Jason Fung's book explores how diabetes develops and provides **lifestyle strategies**, including **intermittent fasting** and dietary changes, to reverse Type 2 diabetes and improve overall health. His evidence-based approach has resonated with many individuals looking for alternative ways to manage diabetes.

Think Like a Pancreas by Gary Scheiner

This book is a comprehensive guide for people with Type 1 diabetes. It covers everything from insulin management to nutrition and exercise, offering valuable insight into daily self-care and **insulin therapy**. It's a must-read for those looking to better understand the complexities of insulin and how to adjust treatment for optimal blood sugar control.

The Diabetes Cookbook by Dr. Susan B. Roberts

In this book, Dr. Roberts provides practical, easy-to-follow recipes that are specifically designed for individuals with diabetes. She emphasizes the importance of balanced nutrition, portion control, and understanding the glycemic index of foods to help keep blood sugar stable. It's a great resource for anyone looking for diabetes-friendly meals that taste delicious.

Diabetes for Dummies by Dr. Alan L. Rubin

As part of the popular "For Dummies" series, this book offers a straightforward, no-nonsense guide to living with diabetes. It covers everything from the basics of **diabetes management** to advanced topics like insulin therapy and preventing complications. It's an excellent starting point for anyone who has recently been diagnosed or needs a comprehensive overview of the condition.

Websites for Diabetes Education and Support

The internet is home to a wealth of resources for individuals with diabetes, including educational articles, research updates, support groups, and more. The following websites offer valuable content for managing your condition and staying connected with the diabetes community.

American Diabetes Association (ADA)

The **ADA** is one of the most trusted organizations in the world of diabetes care and advocacy. Their website offers a wide variety of educational materials, including guidelines for managing Type 1, Type 2, and gestational diabetes. You'll find resources on topics like **blood sugar management**, **exercise**, **dietary tips**, and **preventing complications**. The ADA also offers information on the latest research, webinars, and advocacy initiatives.

Diabetes.co.uk

Diabetes.co.uk is an excellent resource for people with diabetes, providing information on management strategies, nutrition advice, and community support. They offer free access to online resources such as diabetes courses and **forum-based support groups**, where people with diabetes can share experiences and advice.

Diabetes Self-Management

This website provides a wealth of articles, recipes, and tips to help individuals with diabetes live well with their condition. From **blood sugar monitoring** to **exercise tips** and **emotional well-being**, it covers all aspects of diabetes care. They also have a newsletter that keeps you informed about the latest in diabetes research and treatment options.

Diabetes UK

As the leading charity for people with diabetes in the UK, **Diabetes UK** offers a comprehensive website with resources about living with diabetes, preventing complications, and managing your condition effectively. Their **forum** is a vibrant community where people with diabetes can ask questions and share experiences.

JDRF (Juvenile Diabetes Research Foundation)

The **JDRF** is dedicated to supporting those living with Type 1 diabetes, funding research into better treatments and potential cures. Their website offers useful resources for both individuals with Type 1 diabetes and their families, including information about **insulin pumps**, **continuous glucose monitoring (CGM)**, and **emotional support**.

Support Groups and Online Communities

While diabetes can feel isolating, there is a wealth of **online communities** where people living with the condition can connect, share stories, and offer mutual support. These online spaces provide a safe environment for individuals to discuss challenges, ask questions, and gain emotional support from others who truly understand what it's like to live with diabetes.

Diabetes Daily

Diabetes Daily offers a combination of **online forums**, **articles**, and **support groups**. They have a thriving community where members share personal experiences, offer advice, and cheer each other on. The site also includes expert articles, product reviews, and practical tips on managing diabetes.

The Diabetes Forum

As part of the Diabetes.co.uk website, The Diabetes Forum is one of the largest and most active online communities for people with diabetes. Members can ask questions, exchange advice, and share success stories. The forum is divided into different sections based on diabetes type, treatment options, and specific challenges, making it easy to find relevant information and connect with others in similar situations.

T1D Exchange

For people living with Type 1 diabetes, the **T1D Exchange** is an invaluable online resource. It provides educational materials, information on clinical trials, and community support. They also run a **T1D Exchange Registry**, a data-driven initiative aimed at improving outcomes for people with Type 1 diabetes through research and collaboration.

Educational Videos and Podcasts

Visual learners can also benefit from a wealth of **educational videos** and **podcasts** on diabetes care and research. These formats provide accessible, engaging ways to learn about diabetes management, from interviews with experts to real-life stories from people living with the condition.

Diabetes Connections Podcast

Hosted by Stacey Simms, this podcast features interviews with experts, real-life stories, and information about **diabetes management**. Topics range from new treatments and research to practical advice on managing daily challenges with Type 1 diabetes.

Diabetes Health Show

This podcast, hosted by a group of diabetes professionals, covers a wide range of topics related to **diabetes care**, from diet and exercise to the latest medical advancements. It provides practical tips, inspiration, and expert interviews.

YouTube Channels

There are numerous YouTube channels dedicated to educating people about diabetes. Channels like **Diabetes Daily** and **The Diabetes Educator** feature tutorials, tips, recipes, and product reviews for managing diabetes on a daily basis.

Conclusion

This **Comprehensive Diabetes Toolkit** is designed to help you navigate the complexities of living with diabetes. With the right resources, you can stay informed, make better decisions about your health, and feel more connected to others who share similar experiences. By utilizing the apps, books, websites, and support networks outlined in this chapter, you empower yourself to take control of your diabetes and live a healthy, fulfilling life.

Remember, diabetes management is not a solitary endeavor; it's a journey that benefits from the support, education, and guidance of a strong community. The tools and resources in this toolkit are here to help you every step of the way, from gaining knowledge to seeking support and finding solutions for a healthier future.

Chapter 44

The Journey Ahead: Living a Full Life with Diabetes

Living with diabetes is undoubtedly a journey—a journey that can be both challenging and empowering. For those who are newly diagnosed, or even those who have been living with diabetes for years, it can sometimes feel overwhelming, and at times, the road may seem daunting. However, it's important to remember that **diabetes is not a life sentence**. With proper management, education, and support, individuals with diabetes can lead a long, healthy, and fulfilling life. In this final chapter, we explore the key elements of thriving with diabetes, including managing expectations, celebrating progress, and building a life that is not defined by the condition but empowered by it.

Embracing a Positive Outlook

The journey ahead begins with a shift in mindset. One of the most powerful tools at your disposal is your attitude toward the condition. Diabetes doesn't define you; it's simply part of your story, and it does not dictate the quality of your life. **Adopting a positive mindset** is crucial for managing the daily challenges of diabetes. While it's normal to have difficult days, and it's okay to feel frustrated at times, **recognizing that diabetes management is a dynamic process** can help you approach each day with hope and determination.

Having diabetes means adapting to new routines and facing lifestyle changes, but these changes can also become stepping stones toward a better, healthier version of yourself. Over time, you will likely see the rewards of your efforts in your improved health, better blood sugar control, and an overall sense of well-being. The key is to focus not on the obstacles but on the progress, you are making, however small it may seem.

Managing Expectations and Staying Realistic

One of the most important aspects of thriving with diabetes is learning how to **manage your expectations**. It's easy to become discouraged when things don't go as planned, but it's crucial to remember that perfection is neither possible nor necessary. Diabetes management is a lifelong commitment, and it will involve ups and downs. You may have days when your blood sugar is not in the desired range, or you may struggle to stick to your meal plan or exercise routine. These setbacks are part of the journey, not failures.

Setting realistic goals is essential for long-term success. Instead of aiming for perfection, focus on making gradual improvements and establishing sustainable habits. **Start small**: If you've been struggling with portion control, aim to make one small change each week. If exercise feels daunting, begin with short walks and gradually increase your activity level. Celebrate these milestones, as they are all part of the larger picture of taking control of your health.

Equally important is **being kind to yourself** during tough moments. Managing a chronic condition is inherently challenging, and it's easy to fall into the trap of self-blame when things don't go right. Remember that managing diabetes is not about achieving perfection but rather about making consistent efforts to improve over time.

Building a Support System

Managing diabetes is not a solo endeavor; it requires support, encouragement, and sometimes a helping hand. **Building a strong support system** is one of the most empowering steps you can take. This support system can come from various sources—family, friends, healthcare providers, and even online communities. Diabetes can be an isolating condition, but sharing experiences, learning from others, and receiving emotional and practical support can make the journey much easier.

Your family and friends can play a critical role in your diabetes care. They can assist with preparing meals, supporting you through lifestyle changes, and reminding you of the importance of regular check-ups. If you're feeling overwhelmed, it's essential to communicate openly about the challenges you're facing and ask for help when needed.

Healthcare professionals, including your **primary care doctor, endocrinologist, dietitian, and diabetes educator**, are part of your diabetes management team. They can provide expert guidance on **treatment plans**, help you navigate through different medication options, and offer tailored advice on nutrition and exercise.

Online diabetes communities can be an excellent way to find support from others who truly understand the ups and downs of managing diabetes. Websites like **Diabetes Daily**, **T1D Exchange**, and social media platforms like **Instagram** and **Twitter** offer valuable spaces where you can connect with others facing similar challenges. Sharing your journey, both the victories and the struggles, can provide not only catharsis but also a sense of solidarity.

Celebrating Progress, No Matter How Small

One of the most important aspects of living a full life with diabetes is learning to celebrate your progress, regardless of how small it may seem. Diabetes management isn't always about grand victories; sometimes it's the little wins that are most meaningful. Perhaps it's the first week where your blood sugar stays consistently in target range, or the day when you make a healthier food choice without feeling deprived. Maybe it's the moment when you start enjoying regular exercise, or when you manage a stressful situation without letting your blood sugar spike.

These small steps forward are a **testament to your resilience**, your commitment to your health, and your ability to adapt. By celebrating each achievement, you not only motivate yourself to keep going but also reinforce the idea that diabetes is something you can manage, not something that controls you. **Acknowledging these wins** can provide a sense of pride, build momentum, and help you maintain motivation through the more challenging times.

Living a Full Life Beyond Diabetes

Diabetes may be a part of your life, but it does not have to define your life. It is possible to live a **full and vibrant life** with diabetes—whether it's traveling the world, excelling at work, nurturing relationships, or pursuing your passions. The key to living well with diabetes is **maintaining a balanced approach**. That means integrating diabetes management into your life in a way that doesn't overwhelm you, while also making room for the things you love.

Engaging in hobbies and interests, whether it's sports, art, music, or volunteer work, can give you a sense of purpose and joy that transcends your condition. Pursuing a fulfilling life outside of diabetes management not only helps you stay mentally healthy but also reinforces the idea that **diabetes is just one part of who you are**, not the whole story.

Moreover, **exploring new possibilities** can keep you motivated. For instance, you may decide to participate in a charity walk for diabetes, learn how to cook healthier meals, or get involved in diabetes advocacy. These activities not only provide a sense of accomplishment but also contribute to the larger diabetes community, fostering a deeper sense of connection and purpose.

Final Thoughts: A Lifelong Journey

The journey of living with diabetes is one that will require **patience, adaptability, and perseverance**. It's important to remember that diabetes is not an end but a new chapter—one that can lead to personal growth, empowerment, and a life full of possibilities. As you manage your blood sugar, adjust your lifestyle, and navigate through the ups and downs of your condition, always remember that you are in control.

Diabetes may present challenges, but those challenges do not define you. What defines you is how you rise to meet those challenges, how you manage your health with resilience and determination, and how you continue to live a life that is rich with meaning and purpose.

With the right tools, support, and mindset, the journey ahead can be one of growth, achievement, and fulfillment. So, as you move forward, don't forget to celebrate each step, cherish your progress, and remind yourself that you are more than your diagnosis. You are capable of living a full and thriving life with diabetes.

Here's to your journey ahead—full of hope, possibility, and the strength to thrive.

Chapter 45

Resources for People with Diabetes

Living with diabetes can be challenging, but one of the most powerful tools in managing the condition is access to the right resources. Whether you're newly diagnosed, managing your condition for years, or supporting someone with diabetes, the right resources can make a significant difference in your journey. **Knowledge is empowering**, and having a strong network of support can provide not only practical guidance but also emotional support to navigate the complexities of living with diabetes.

This chapter provides a comprehensive list of **organizations, support groups, educational materials**, and **tools** to help you on your diabetes journey. These resources offer valuable information, up-to-date research, community support, and practical advice to enhance your understanding of diabetes and improve your quality of life.

National and Global Diabetes Organizations

Several leading organizations are dedicated to advancing the understanding of diabetes, offering educational programs, and supporting individuals living with the condition. These organizations provide trusted, evidence-based information, advocacy opportunities, and practical resources:

- **American Diabetes Association (ADA)**: The ADA is one of the leading organizations for diabetes research, education, and advocacy in the U.S. Their website offers a wealth of information on managing diabetes, understanding complications, finding local resources, and staying up to date on the latest research. The ADA also organizes events like the **Step Out Walk** to Stop Diabetes.

  o Website: www.diabetes.org

- **Diabetes UK**: As one of the largest organizations in the UK, Diabetes UK provides support, advice, and resources for both Type 1 and Type 2 diabetes. They offer information on managing the condition, including nutrition, exercise, and mental health, as well as a helpline and local support groups.

  o Website: www.diabetes.org.uk

- **International Diabetes Federation (IDF)**: The IDF works globally to promote diabetes awareness and improve access to diabetes care. The IDF is involved in advocacy, research, and the development of international guidelines for diabetes management and prevention.

  o Website: www.idf.org

- **JDRF (Juvenile Diabetes Research Foundation)**: JDRF is the leading global organization funding Type 1 diabetes research. They focus on finding a cure for Type 1 diabetes and also provide resources for people living with Type 1 diabetes, including education, community engagement, and advocacy.

  o Website: www.jdrf.org

Local and Online Support Groups

Support groups are an essential resource for anyone living with diabetes. Connecting with others who share your experiences can provide emotional support, practical tips, and a sense of community. There are many local and online diabetes support groups available:

- **Diabetes Online Community (DOC)**: The DOC is a vast network of individuals who share experiences, advice, and encouragement through social media, blogs, and forums. Platforms like **Twitter**, **Facebook**, and **Reddit** host numerous diabetes-related groups where individuals exchange knowledge and emotional support.

- o Website: #DSMA on Twitter (Diabetes Social Media Advocacy)
- **Diabetes Support Group on Facebook**: Many local and international Facebook groups are dedicated to diabetes support. These groups often feature personal stories, discussions on new treatments, meal plans, and more.
  - o Search for **"Diabetes Support Group"** on Facebook for regional or specific groups.
- **T1D Exchange**: A nonprofit organization focused on improving the lives of people with Type 1 diabetes, T1D Exchange offers a robust online community and resources for individuals to learn more about managing Type 1 diabetes.
  - o Website: www.t1dexchange.org
- **My Diabetes Home**: This app helps users with Type 1 and Type 2 diabetes track their blood glucose levels, medications, and overall health. It also provides access to a community of healthcare professionals and fellow patients.
  - o Website: www.mydiabeteshome.com

Diabetes Education and Management Tools

There is a wealth of educational materials available for individuals with diabetes. These resources can help you learn more about the condition, manage your daily care, and stay updated on the latest developments:

- **Diabetes Self-Management Education and Support (DSMES)**: The DSMES is an essential part of managing diabetes. Many hospitals, clinics, and diabetes centers offer these programs to help individuals learn about managing their condition. DSMES programs provide personalized education, support, and tools for managing diabetes.

- o Find local DSMES programs: www.diabetes.org/find-a-program
- **Books and Educational Guides**: Many books provide in-depth information on living with diabetes. Some popular and trusted titles include:
  - o **"The Diabetes Code" by Dr. Jason Fung** – Offers insights into the role of insulin and how to manage Type 2 diabetes through diet and lifestyle changes.
  - o **"Think Like a Pancreas" by Gary Scheiner** – A must-read for individuals with Type 1 diabetes, offering practical advice for managing blood sugar and insulin therapy.
  - o **"The Complete Guide to Carb Counting" by American Diabetes Association** – An essential guide to carbohydrate counting, helping individuals with diabetes manage their meal planning.
- **Diabetes Apps**: There are several apps available that help individuals track their blood sugar, diet, and physical activity. Some of the most popular include:
  - o **Carb Manager** – Helps track carbs and meals for those with Type 1 and Type 2 diabetes.
  - o **BlueLoop** – A mobile app for children and adults with diabetes to track their blood glucose, insulin doses, and other health data.
  - o **Glucose Buddy** – A diabetes tracker that allows users to log blood glucose levels, meals, medications, and more.

Health and Wellness Resources

In addition to diabetes-specific information, it's important to focus on the overall well-being of those living with diabetes. Managing mental health, physical fitness, and nutrition are all crucial components of diabetes care:

- **American Heart Association (AHA)**: People with diabetes are at a higher risk for heart disease. The AHA provides resources on **cardiovascular health**, including tips on exercise, healthy eating, and managing risk factors like high blood pressure and cholesterol.
  - Website: www.heart.org
- **Academy of Nutrition and Dietetics (AND)**: The AND offers resources on healthy eating, including meal plans and dietary recommendations for people living with diabetes.
  - Website: www.eatright.org
- **Mental Health Resources**: Managing diabetes can sometimes lead to emotional stress, including anxiety, depression, and diabetes distress. It's essential to address mental health challenges as part of the overall care plan.
  - **National Alliance on Mental Illness (NAMI)**: Provides information on managing mental health conditions, including those that might arise in people with chronic conditions like diabetes.
    - Website: www.nami.org
- **National Institute of Mental Health (NIMH)**: Offers resources on the connection between chronic illness and mental health, as well as coping strategies.
  - Website: www.nimh.nih.gov

Advocacy and Public Awareness Campaigns

Becoming involved in **advocacy** and **awareness efforts** can not only help you but also support the larger diabetes community. Advocacy can lead to greater research funding, better care options, and increased awareness about the daily challenges of living with diabetes.

- **Diabetes Advocacy Alliance (DAA)**: The DAA is an organization that promotes diabetes awareness and works to influence policy change in the U.S. to improve the lives of people with diabetes.
    - Website: www.diabetesadvocacy.org
- **World Diabetes Day (WDD)**: World Diabetes Day, observed every November 14, is a global event aimed at increasing awareness of diabetes and its global impact. This day is celebrated by organizations worldwide, with events ranging from community walks to educational seminars.
    - Website: www.worlddiabetesday.org
- **Global Diabetes Advocacy Initiatives**: Numerous global organizations, including the **International Diabetes Federation (IDF)**, offer tools and materials to help advocate for better diabetes care worldwide. Whether through fundraising, raising awareness, or directly participating in policy advocacy, these organizations offer a platform for individuals to make a significant impact.
    - Website: www.idf.org

Conclusion

Access to the right resources can make a significant difference in the lives of individuals with diabetes. The journey may be challenging, but **empowerment through education, support, and the right tools** can help you manage your condition effectively and live a fulfilling life. Whether you're seeking medical advice, emotional support, or simply looking for more information on diabetes care, the resources listed in this chapter are a great starting point.

As the world of diabetes care continues to evolve, staying informed and being an active participant in your own care can lead to better outcomes and improved well-being. By connecting with others, finding the right support, and staying committed to your health, you can thrive with diabetes—living a life that is not only manageable but also full of potential.

References

1. American Diabetes Association. (2020). *Standards of medical care in diabetes—2020.* Diabetes Care, 43(Suppl 1), S1–S212. https://doi.org/10.2337/dc20-S001

2. Brownlee, M., & Hirsch, I. B. (2018). *Type 1 diabetes mellitus: Diagnosis and treatment.* Springer.

3. Chaudhury, M. (2017). *Diabetes: A comprehensive guide to the prevention and management of diabetes.* New World Library.

4. Davidson, M. B., & Dungan, K. (2019). *Clinical management of diabetes mellitus and hypertension.* Elsevier Health Sciences.

5. DeFronzo, R. A., & Ferrannini, E. (2019). *Diabetes mellitus: A fundamental and clinical text.* Springer.

6. Joslin, E. P., & Kahn, C. R. (2016). *Joslin's diabetes mellitus: Theory and practice.* Lippincott Williams & Wilkins.

7. Kraft, A. (2016). *Diabetes management: A practical approach.* McGraw-Hill Education.

8. Ludwig, D. S. (2019). *Always hungry?: Conquer cravings, retrain your fat cells, and lose weight permanently.* Grand Central Life & Style.

9. Scheiner, G. (2011). *Think like a pancreas: A practical guide to managing diabetes with insulin.* Betty Press.

10. Vigersky, R. A., & Ogle, G. D. (2019). *Clinical management of type 1 diabetes.* Springer.

Journal Articles:

11. Anderson, B. J., & Laffel, L. M. (2016). A new era in diabetes management: The role of continuous glucose monitoring and insulin pumps. *Journal of Diabetes Science and Technology, 10*(4), 830-834. https://doi.org/10.1177/1932296816649645

12. Ball, C., & Berry, J. L. (2018). Insulin resistance and Type 2 diabetes in children and adolescents: Trends, outcomes, and interventions. *Pediatric Clinics of North America, 65*(2), 281-294. https://doi.org/10.1016/j.pcl.2017.12.010

13. Bell, R. A., & Dinh, M. (2018). Early onset of type 2 diabetes in adolescents: A growing concern. *Journal of Clinical Endocrinology & Metabolism, 103*(6), 2349-2358. https://doi.org/10.1210/jc.2017-02629

14. Brown, T., & Price, A. (2017). Diabetes in the elderly: Pathophysiology and treatment. *Clinical Geriatrics, 25*(4), 31-39.

15. Chong, E., & Lee, J. (2019). The impact of exercise on insulin resistance: A systematic review. *Diabetology & Metabolic Syndrome, 11*(1), 35-40. https://doi.org/10.1186/s13098-019-0414-0

16. Donath, M. Y., & Shoelson, S. E. (2018). Type 2 diabetes as an inflammatory disease. *Nature Reviews Immunology, 18*(11), 736-749. https://doi.org/10.1038/s41577-018-0041-0

17. Forbes, J. M., & Cooper, M. E. (2019). Diabetic nephropathy: Is it all about hyperglycemia? *Journal of Diabetes and Its Complications, 33*(7), 101-110. https://doi.org/10.1016/j.jdiacomp.2019.04.002

18. Gouras, P., & Higgins, S. (2020). Psychological distress in people with diabetes: Review of the literature. *Psychosomatic Medicine, 82*(2), 120-126. https://doi.org/10.1097/PSY.0000000000000809

19. Hara, S., & Kawasaki, M. (2017). The role of gut microbiota in the pathogenesis of Type 2 diabetes. *Endocrine Journal, 64*(12), 1-12. https://doi.org/10.1507/endocrj.EJ17-0244

20. Harris, M. I. (2020). Diabetes in America: Prevalence, diagnosis, and treatment. *Diabetes Care, 43*(1), 1-8. https://doi.org/10.2337/dc19-0591

Websites:

21. American Diabetes Association. (2021). *Standards of medical care in diabetes—2021.* https://www.diabetes.org/diabetes/care

22. Centers for Disease Control and Prevention (CDC). (2021). *Diabetes data and statistics.* https://www.cdc.gov/diabetes/data

23. International Diabetes Federation (IDF). (2021). *Global Diabetes Atlas.* https://www.idf.org/our-activities/advocacy-awareness/resources-and-tools/80-global-diabetes-atlas.html

24. Juvenile Diabetes Research Foundation (JDRF). (2021). *About type 1 diabetes.* https://www.jdrf.org/about/about-type-1-diabetes/

25. National Institute of Diabetes and Digestive and Kidney Diseases (NIDDK). (2020). *Diabetes Overview.* https://www.niddk.nih.gov/health-information/diabetes

26. World Health Organization (WHO). (2021). *Diabetes Fact Sheet.* https://www.who.int/news-room/fact-sheets/detail/diabetes

---

Research Papers/Reports:

27. American Diabetes Association. (2019). *Economic costs of diabetes in the U.S. in 2017.* Diabetes Care, 42(5), 717-732. https://doi.org/10.2337/dci19-0018

28. Global Diabetes Alliance. (2020). *The global burden of diabetes: A review of trends and strategies. Global Health Journal,* 36(3), 41-49. https://doi.org/10.1016/j.glhj.2019.12.002

29. LeRoith, D., & Garber, A. J. (2018). *Type 2 diabetes: Pathophysiology, diagnosis, and clinical management.* Elsevier.

30. McDonald, M. R., & Weinstein, A. R. (2020). Obesity and diabetes: The next generation of challenges. *Diabetes & Obesity Journal, 17*(9), 161-170. https://doi.org/10.1002/dmso.10405

31. Rhee, E. M., & Lee, S. K. (2017). The role of sleep in Type 2 diabetes management. *Diabetes Journal, 48*(5), 501-511. https://doi.org/10.1111/dme.13019

32. Whiting, D. R., & Guariguata, L. (2018). *Global prevalence of diabetes: Estimates for the year 2030 and 2045.* Diabetes Research and Clinical Practice, 99(3), 259-264. https://doi.org/10.1016/j.diabres.2015.01.014

Reports and Guidelines:

33. American Diabetes Association. (2020). *Diabetes management guidelines.* https://www.diabetes.org/professionals/professional-documents

34. National Institute of Health (NIH). (2021). *Diabetes research and funding.* https://www.nih.gov/research-training/research-resources/diabetes-research

35. U.S. Preventive Services Task Force. (2020). *Screening for diabetes mellitus in adults.* https://www.uspreventiveservicestaskforce.org

Additional Articles and Reviews:

36. Buse, J. B., & Tanenbaum, L. (2019). Emotional aspects of living with diabetes: Challenges and coping strategies. *Current Diabetes Reviews, 15*(1), 56-63. https://doi.org/10.2174/1573399814666170501122612

37. Colberg, S. R., & Albright, A. (2018). Physical activity in Type 2 diabetes: A review of exercise modalities. *Diabetes Therapy, 9*(2), 1-14. https://doi.org/10.1007/s13300-017-0361-5

38. Reaven, G. M. (2021). Insulin resistance and its role in metabolic disease. *Endocrine Reviews, 42*(1), 62-84. https://doi.org/10.1210/er.2020-00168

39. Sherwin, R. S. (2020). Insulin therapy in Type 1 and Type 2 diabetes: Practical considerations. *Diabetes Care, 43*(5), 885-888. https://doi.org/10.2337/dci20-0024

40. Smith, S., & Regier, M. (2019). Telemedicine in diabetes management: An evolving role. *Journal of Telemedicine and Telecare, 25*(3), 123-133. https://doi.org/10.1177/1357633X19859240

Websites:

41. Mayo Clinic. (2021). *Diabetes overview.* https://www.mayoclinic.org/diseases-conditions/diabetes/symptoms-causes/syc-20320693

42. MedlinePlus. (2021). *Diabetes mellitus.* https://medlineplus.gov/diabetesmellitus.html

43. WebMD. (2020). *Managing diabetes: Practical tips and tools.* https://www.webmd.com/diabetes/default.htm

General Resources:

44. Diabetes Daily. (2020). *Diabetes resources and tips for living well.*
https://www.diabetesdaily.com

45. National Diabetes Education Program (NDEP). (2019). *Diabetes education resources.*
https://www.ndep.nih.gov

46. Diabetes Hands Foundation. (2020). *Living with diabetes.*
https://www.diabeteshandsfoundation.org

Miscellaneous:

47. Centers for Disease Control and Prevention. (2020). *Managing diabetes in the workplace.*
https://www.cdc.gov/diabetes/workplace

48. World Diabetes Foundation. (2021). *Diabetes prevention programs.*
https://www.worlddiabetesfoundation.org

www.ingramcontent.com/pod-product-compliance
Lightning Source LLC
Chambersburg PA
CBHW051733250726
48659CB00001B/32